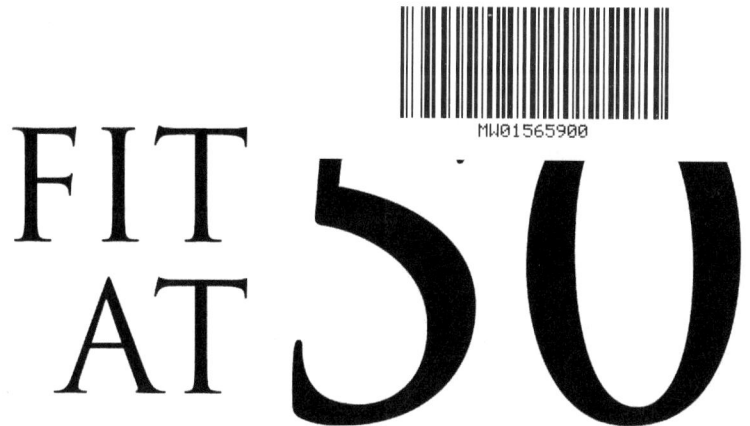

FIT AT 50

BACK FROM THE BRINK, NATURALLY

Matthew McLaughlin

outskirtspress
DENVER, COLORADO

The opinions expressed in this manuscript are solely the opinions of the author and do not represent the opinions or thoughts of the publisher. The author has represented and warranted full ownership and/or legal right to publish all the materials in this book.

Fit at 50: Back From the Brink, Naturally
All Rights Reserved.
Copyright © 2013 Matthew McLaughlin
v4.0

© 2013 Cover Photo by Felicty Murphy. All rights reserved - used with permission.

This book may not be reproduced, transmitted, or stored in whole or in part by any means, including graphic, electronic, or mechanical without the express written consent of the publisher except in the case of brief quotations embodied in critical articles and reviews.

Outskirts Press, Inc.
http://www.outskirtspress.com

ISBN: 978-1-4327-9241-1

Library of Congress Control Number: 2012946787

Outskirts Press and the "OP" logo are trademarks belonging to Outskirts Press, Inc.

PRINTED IN THE UNITED STATES OF AMERICA

Acknowledgments

First, I must thank my mother for the endless hours she spent with me, helping me learn to read. As her only child with dyslexia, we became very close, in part from the substantial amount of time she spent sitting beside me on the couch as I struggled to read. I must also thank mom and my dad, God rest his soul, for having given me a good set of genetics to work with. My goal is to waste none of them.

I must also thank Physical Therapist Robert "Bob" Forster for being patient but persistent with me through the years, until I accepted his recommendation to use periodization. Through the years he has been a constant guide and in that time, he has also become a good friend. He has healed tens of thousands of injured people, allowing them to get back to doing the things they love. A byproduct of his physical therapy practice has been the creation of an extensive knowledge base which documents the actions which cause injury. He uses this information to help others by providing many free seminars each year in which he lectures on how to avoid injury. He has guided me, and many others, with this information which has allowed me to continue my "athletic career" at a level well above and beyond what would have been possible otherwise.

I would like to thank Bob's staff at Forster Physical Therapy and Phase IV, and particularly Exercise Physiologist Aishea Mass. With the treatment they have provided, they have let me continue to do many of the things I love. Aishea has also been a long-term sounding board as I have sorted out many of the physiological principals detailed in this book.

I must also thank Robert Portman, PhD; Andrew Mikaelian, MD; Linda Gerrits, MD; Exercise Physiologist Aishea Mass; and Robert Forster PT, for reviewing all or part of the manuscript and providing feedback to ensure the concepts are conveyed as correctly as possible.

I also need to thank photographer Felicity Murphy for the wonderful images on the covers and in the book, as she made this old man look presentable. I also want to thank hairstylist Karissa Dawson for giving me a great cut every time.

I would also like to mention a word about the charity "Pearls of Hope" which is on my race kit and will receive a portion of the proceeds from every book I sell. George Jackson and I became friends after meeting on the Santa Ana Community College track team, and we are dear friends to this day. He would eventually meet and marry a wonderful woman, Lorraine Jackson. Lorraine would eventually contract and survive breast cancer. Some years ago she created the Lorraine Jackson Foundation and the "Pearls of Hope" charity, which provides college scholarships to children who have lost parents to breast cancer. Nearly 40,000 women die from breast cancer in the US each year. Please help Lorraine provide more scholarships to more deserving children by donating at least 1 dollar to Pearls of Hope each year for every pound you lose by following the recommendations in this book.

Above all, I want to thank my wonderful wife and daughters for allowing me to take the time to write this. I also want to thank them for being the best part of my life.

Contents

    Introduction xi
1. Life Is About Balance. 1
2. About the Author 9
3. Periodization or Something Else 22
4. Mechanics of Running 35
5. Mechanics of Cycling 43
6. Mechanics of Freestyle Swimming 48
7. Getting a Coach 51
8. Motivation 53
9. Injury Prevention 56
10. Perceived vs. Actual Exertion 60
11. BLT vs VO2 MAX 62
12. Tailoring Your Program 66
13. Stretching 67
14. Strength Training 76
15. Hydration 111
16. Post-Workout and Race Nutrition 116
17. Eating Program 118
18. Starting Your Cardiovascular Program 132
19. Getting Started on the Bike 142
20. Getting Started Swimming 147
21. Logging 151
22. Final Word 153
    Appendix A 155
    References 159

Foreword BY ROBERT FORSTER, PT

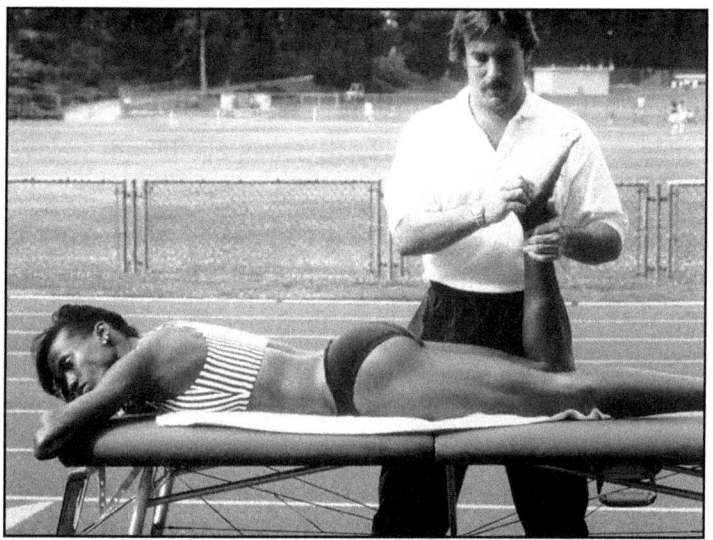

Photo by: John Livzey

Above, Physical Therapist Bob Forster is working on Jackie Joyner-Kersee in preparation for the Barcelona Olympic Games in 1992 where she would win Gold again in the Heptathlon. At the time of this publishing, she still held the World Record in the Heptathlon, a record she set at the Seoul Olympic Games in 1988, making it one of the longest-standing World Records ever. Jackie is one of the many Olympians and World Record-setting athletes Bob has helped over the years.

"After 20 years of practicing physical therapy, I founded Phase IV Scientific Health and Performance Centers in 2002 to address the needs of the growing number of highly competitive age group athletes in a variety of endurance sports. The genesis of this new science-based training center came from my desire to share the knowledge gained working with some of the most successful coaches in the results-driven arena of elite and professional athletics. While still working with professional athletes, our primary goal is to provide amateur athletes with the latest scientific training methodologies to match their intense desire to reach their highest genetic potential, injury-free. In a world full of hype, fads, and gimmicks, the amateur has had access to little more than the information found in lay press periodicals to solve the roadblocks to personal athletic achievement. At Phase IV, there are no gurus other than science!

The foundation of all science-based training is an assessment of the physiological adaptations that must be achieved to perform at the highest level for a given athlete in a specific event. The training program must be designed to methodically foster those adaptations through the manipulation of training volume and intensity over the course of months and years.

When training elite athletes, there are specific predetermined goals to be achieved in each phase of training. The goals of each phase are based on an understanding of the scientifically rational sequence of fitness and skill development, and a calculation of the physiological requirements needed to win. Satisfy the goals, check the box, and move toward a peak by building on the foundation laid in each previous phase of training.

What I have experienced in amateur athletes is the urge to train harder and harder, stopping only when they are injured or overtrained. Instead of patience and an understanding of the need to develop each aspect of fitness for its inherent value toward peak fitness, there is a tendency to train aimlessly and aggressively toward their goals.

For the master's level athlete this approach is especially detrimental as there are well-documented declines in the ability to recover from workouts in direct relation to decreasing hormone production with age. The mature athlete is also more likely to have limitations on their time to train, which further requires the need to train smarter, not harder.

When I met Matt he was one of those struggling amateurs trying to find the answers, but equipped with only the basic knowledge gained from competing in high school and college athletics, and an inquiring mind. When first introduced to the science of periodization training he was doubtful, and apt to relapse into his old way of thinking. It took a few humbling setbacks for him to realize there is a better way to train and achieve his goals. Since that time, Matt has not only solved his roadblocks and achieved athletic success on a national level, but he has helped many others along the way as he preached the principles of scientific training.

The science he has followed successfully for years, and shared with so many of the athletes he has coached, he now presents here as an easy-to-understand and inspiring account of his journey using science-based training to reach the highest levels of performance. For me, this book is the realization of my goal to pass on the science-based training methodologies used by the pros to the people who have the heart and desire to reach their potential but previously lacked the guidance provided by sound science. Follow the science and you too will find the perfect coach and training partner to achieve your athletic dreams."

Introduction

CONSULT A PHYSICIAN BEFORE STARTING THIS OR ANY FITNESS program. I want you to see a physician and get a complete physical before you start so you can identify and treat any existing issues. You will also need your doctor's help to identify any areas of this program you should tailor to your specific needs or sensitivities. I also want you to see your physician to establish a baseline so you can measure your progress. Staying motivated is a big part of any fitness program, and seeing progress is one of the most powerful motivators. What you can expect from this program is to look better on the outside and feel better on the inside as a result of improved health. The best way to measure fitness and health improvements is to get a complete physical every year.

Also, because I work for the FBI, and had to get permission from the FBI to publish this book, the FBI wants me to clarify that the opinions in this book are mine and not the FBI's.

This book is meant to serve as a complete, yet simple guide to global health and fitness. Global health and fitness are about balance, in your training program and in life. A balanced fitness program is one that fits into the rest of your life. I am a devoted husband and father, and a dedicated professional. Over the last decade I have developed this fitness program to be a part of a well-balanced life.

I must also point out that it is not possible to attain any real fitness with only 10 or 20 minutes a day. There are a lot of programs which depend on hype to sell you whatever fad exercise routine or piece of equipment they think you will buy that day. Those programs are not telling you the truth. While doing 10 minutes of anything may be better than doing nothing at all, the suggestion that you can attain a reasonable level of fitness in that small amount of time is simply not true.

There are also no magic pills, literally. You see a lot of ads touting pills you should take or a substance you can sprinkle on your food to lose weight. In many cases, there are side effects which can be very dangerous, and in the long run could harm you. Even if they help you lose a pound or two, is the idea to use them for the rest of your life to control your weight?

The better option is to understand how your body works and make a few adjustments in several areas to safely lose weight and improve your fitness and health. This book is a simple, easy-to-follow guide in all these areas. The reality is, you should expect to spend about an hour a day to attain total health and fitness.

I put in at least 50 hours a week at work and still attend most school and other events involving my wife and daughters. I have also coached my daughters' soccer and track teams, and still manage to workout an average of about 1 hour and 15 minutes a day. I have a couple of National Championships I am chasing and the level of competition in this country requires me to spend a little more time to get to my genetic potential. But that is driven by my goals. Your goals starting out should be simply to improve health and fitness. Once you have reached that goal, then it will be time to reassess and determine whether your commitment to yourself and your new fitness and health goals require some adjustments. You will need to be a little selfish to take time each day to improve your health and fitness. However, in doing so, you can make every aspect of your life better. Through weight loss, an increase in muscle mass, and improved blood flow resulting from a better cardiovascular exercise program, everything will change for the better.

1. LIFE IS ABOUT BALANCE.

FIT AT 50: BACK FROM THE BRINK, NATURALLY IS THE STORY OF A lifetime athlete who almost lost the ability to do something he loved: compete. Like most athletes of my generation I had learned to train and compete through pain. When in school, training through pain was a test of manhood and teamwork. After graduating from college, training and racing in pain was a habit, and the worst kind. When I entered my 30s, ignoring pain usually meant I was ignoring an injury, which was causing the pain, so by continuing to train and race I made the injuries worse. The only reason I eventually sought medical care and physical therapy was because I couldn't continue. My body was breaking down in several areas at one time. I was at the brink of athletic oblivion.

I had to either stop training and racing, or change how I was doing those things. Since I enjoyed being fit and racing, I decided to finally listen to my physical therapist, Bob Forster, one of the foremost physical therapists in the country, who had been telling me for years about the program I needed to adopt. Bob and a great orthopedic surgeon would put me on the right track. To get there, I would have to undergo surgery for a shoulder injury, be patient during physical therapy, and then learn a new training system, called periodization.

I made the changes 10 years ago, at age 42, and have suffered only a few minor injuries since. I learned my lessons well and began listening to my body. I learned to identify issue areas and treat them early, before they became injuries. This involved some self-treatment, which meant doing some deep tissue massage and icing.

These new skills allowed me to treat myself when muscles were just tight, before they became actual injuries.

What is in the pages that follow are the lessons learned about the complex human body, but in the most distilled form possible. Fitness can be confusing because of its complexity and the amount of information out there, much of which is contradictory.

What I have done in this book is very similar to the vetting process I went through as a polygraph examiner. When I graduated polygraph school in 1987, I was taught that most polygraph examinations should take three to four hours. During the six years I was a polygraph examiner for the Naval Investigative Service, now known as Naval Investigative Criminal Service (NCIS), and the two years as a polygraph examiner with the FBI, I determined that many of the complex explanations I had been told were necessary to conduct a successful polygraph examination were in fact unnecessary.

Although it was important for me to know everything they taught me about physiology, over time I figured out that some of what I was explaining to examinees when preparing them to be tested was actually increasing their anxiety. Increased anxiety resulted in less focus by the examinee on what was important: the test questions themselves.

I began evaluating each part of how I explained the test, and then started tailoring or eliminating material. After eight years, I had boiled the explanation for a pre-employment screening examination down to about 30 minutes, with the entire test running about 1 hour and 15 minutes. I would take substantially longer if it was an examination regarding a criminal matter. This was necessary to establish good rapport with the examinee, so if he or she failed the test the ground work was laid for an interrogation.

I have done the same thing regarding health and fitness, and this book is the result of a thorough vetting process. There is a tremendous amount of information today about fitness and health. The art of becoming and remaining healthy and fit, while being a good husband and father and also maintaining a demanding career, forced me to develop and use highly effective and efficient health and fitness strategies.

This book is intended to be a comprehensive guide regarding the commitments you will need to make to yourself to bring change. It is also possible to employ in stages the various strategies in the pages that follow. For instance, if you can't make time for the strength training or cardio programs, then start with just the eating program and start stretching every day. Then, after you've lost a few pounds and decide you want to fit another part of the program into your life, get a gym membership and start doing some strength or cardio training, or both.

How dramatic your end results are will be determined by how committed you are to yourself and to this program.

To begin, get a complete physical so you can identify any health issue you might need to be concerned with or accommodate. Once you get clearance from your doctor to start this program, as additional motivation, take a "before" photo. It's always easier to press forward when you see how far you have come.

Gradual Change Is the Best Change

This program is radically different from the routines I used in high school and college. It is smart, simple, and complete. In the pages that follow, you will find the tools to turn the clock back. As a result of the complexity of the human body, meaningful changes won't happen overnight, but if you can be patient, once they occur they will be lasting.

This is a global program, which simply illustrates a proper eating program that allows you to eat like a man (or woman), not a mouse, which means you will still eat most or all of your favorite foods and still lose weight. Part of what makes my eating program sustainable is that it focuses on moderation, not deprivation.

Perhaps the best news is that the eating program is likely very similar to the way you eat now. This means you will likely not have to radically change what you eat and drink. You may need to modify your portions and place certain foods in different parts of the day, compared to how you eat now. But, by using this program, you will lose weight and develop a faster metabolism, especially if you start exercising the right way.

By becoming more fit, and understanding what different foods do, you will eventually be able to eat more of your favorite foods and still remain fit. This will happen as a result of an increase in muscle mass, which speeds up your metabolism, so you will burn more calories, even at rest.

This program also provides simple guidance regarding proper cardiovascular training, strength training, and stretching. It will give you the tools to become leaner, stronger, and faster through better mobility and functional strength.

I must point out that when I talk about increased muscle mass, you don't need to worry about becoming musclebound, for several reasons. One, the strength training in this program is designed to increase functional strength and does not focus on just building big "show" muscles. Additionally, people who become musclebound usually spend many hours a day lifting weights, and may also take dangerous and even illegal supplements.

I spend about two hours a week on strength training. I use lighter weights than I used to and execute very precise movements in the right sequence to attain functional strength. Through the use of the many exercises detailed in the strength training section, and a periodized schedule, I have naturally increased my production of beneficial hormones, like testosterone. Coupled with a proper eating program, I am in the best shape of my life, and you can be too.

This program is about using the body's natural ability to get stronger and function better, internally and externally. This program will bring positive changes, more slowly than some other programs, but they can last a lifetime.

When I started using the program I stopped getting injured, and started getting stronger and faster. Colleagues began asking what I was doing differently. I explained the workout program I had started using. Several of them started using the program and saw similar results. The program works because it takes advantage of the body's natural ability to adapt.

When I started using the program I used it for running only. Then, after having shoulder surgery, I applied it to all of my strength training and saw benefits there too. Then, at age 49, I found the sport of triathlon and applied the program to swimming and biking and saw great results there as well.

As a living case study and having coached many athletes for nearly a decade, I know this program works. This program is different from most others because it promotes gradual improvement. Gradual improvement is the best, because it is the safest and most sustainable. There are a lot of programs out there which, in some cases, can help you achieve fast results. The problem with these gimmick programs is that they are typically not sustainable because of their extremely high intensity. In some cases, they may be great to jump start a fitness program, but they can easily lead to injury, especially for those who are older or not already fit.

WHY BE FIT?

The American Heritage Stedman's Medical Dictionary defines fitness as: "The state or condition of being physically sound and healthy, especially as the result of exercise and proper nutrition." The benefits of better fitness are many, starting with a better life by reducing the chance of a number of severe health conditions, such as heart disease, stroke, high blood pressure, diabetes, and Alzheimer's, to name a few. A proper fitness program, which includes strength training, also helps prevent or combat conditions such as osteoporosis and sarcopenia. Osteoporosis refers to a loss of bone density, and sarcopenia refers to a loss of muscle mass. Proper strength training fights both of these conditions. As your strength improves through an increase in muscle mass, tendons and ligaments get stronger. This causes your bones to adapt and become more dense.

After age 30, people who are inactive will lose at least 3 to 5 percent of their muscle mass every 10 years. This condition is called sarcopenia. This loss of muscle mass parallels a reduction of testosterone production, which peaks at around age 30. This reduction in muscle mass also contributes to a weakening of tendons and ligaments, which leads to a loss of bone density. This condition is problematic in another way. The reduction of muscle mass slows the metabolism. Combine a slower metabolism with the typical decrease in physical activity for most Americans, and the fat creeps on. By age 50, the average American male has lost a lot of muscle and put on 20 to 40 pounds of fat. The good news is, there is a cure: strength training.

This program not only focuses on skeletal muscular fitness, which will result in a natural increase of testosterone production and help fight sarcopenia and osteoporosis, but also on the most important muscle in the body: your heart. When both areas are improved, your metabolism speeds up and your heart gets stronger, resulting in an increase in blood flow throughout your body. Combine this with a proper eating program and you can create lasting positive change. This also means, when you get to the fitness level you want, you will be able to eat a little more and still maintain your weight.

I used the eating program in this book four years ago to lose about 10 pounds, and I did it without changing my training schedule. I didn't lose any weight the first two weeks. But, the third week I lost half a pound and continued to lose at that rate until I lost all

LIFE IS ABOUT BALANCE.

10 pounds. Then, when I started triathlon training and started swimming and riding my bike a couple of times a week, I lost two more pounds, putting me at 165. I then lost another couple of pounds, but that weight loss put me at a number below what I weighed in high school. That was too lean and I started to lose some strength. To solve the problem, I had to actually increase my calorie intake and did so by "carbohydrate loading" each night before bed. I put the two pounds back on, and my strength returned, establishing my race weight.

One of the keys to any successful fitness program is setting goals. Goals are important in life. We need things to look forward to so we can work toward them. The key to setting goals is making sure they are attainable. If your goal is weight loss, it is fine to have a distant goal of the total you want to lose. However, the key in setting weight-loss goals is to set the initial goal so you can attain it in a few months. So, a near-term weight loss goal should be to lose five pounds in four to six weeks. When you have achieved that goal, you will know that what you are doing works, and be even more resolute to lose more weight. The next goal should be to lose another five pounds, and so on, until you have reached your long- term target weight.

A couple of years, after urging from myself and his wife, my good friend got a physical. The doctor determined his blood pressure and cholesterol were a little high and he had two choices: either lose 20 pounds or start taking medication. He decided to lose the weight, did, and then never needed the medication.

Not only can better fitness lead to a longer better life, it can also lower health care costs. Four years ago, I applied for a new life insurance policy. One condition of the application was that I had to get a physical. My wife was surprised when she received the policy quote. As a result of my fitness level, the cost of the coverage was much lower than she expected.

So, if we agree that life is about balance, we should also agree that as we progress we will need to re-balance, since the rest of life will keep changing while you become more fit and healthy. Some people treat their own personal health and fitness like they treat the weather: they talk about it but they never do anything about it. It is your body, your fitness, your health -- and you can have a positive impact on all of them if you set realistic goals, have a good program, and then commit. No one else can do this for you; you must do it yourself.

Gandhi said: "You must be the change you wish to see in the world."

2. About the Author

I BEGAN RUNNING TRACK WHEN I WAS NINE. A LEADER WITH THE Santa Ana Parks and Recreation Department saw me running around the playground at school and asked me if I wanted to run track. He was a track coach. I said, "I don't know. What do you do in track?" He said, "You get to run against other kids in races." That sounded like fun, and so began my athletic career.

I was one of the fastest kids at my elementary school and I was pretty coordinated, too. I was drawn to sports at this early age, in part because of the struggles I experienced in the classroom from dyslexia.

Spelling and reading were nightmares for me. My biggest fan and supporter, my mom, spent endless hours sitting next to me on the couch in the living room helping me to read. At one point she exploited my very large sweet tooth. When I became highly frustrated and ready to stop reading, she induced me to keep going by giving me a Hershey's Kiss. She was teaching me to keep reading, keep fighting.

Dyslexia is a developmental reading disorder that occurs when the brain does not properly recognize certain symbols or the order of the symbols, usually when reading. It is as though the signal sent from the eye is disrupted en route to the brain for translation. At first glance, I might read the word "stop" as "pots." To overcome this, one must "manually" force the brain to reconcile these images so the message on the page can be translated and understood clearly. This requires a tremendous amount of energy, and accounts for why even today I am able to read only one chapter or so at a time before becoming fatigued.

In school, my greatest frustration was having to read or spell a difficult word out loud. Even in a high school English class, I remember reading out loud a story, which contained the word "fatigue." It was the first time I had seen the word, so I pronounced it phonetically: fat-i-gue instead of: fa-teeg. What had haunted me in grade school followed, a burble of laughter through the class causing me to turn bright red from embarrassment. To this day I am still a poor speller and slow reader, but I manage.

As I look back, my struggle with dyslexia, like any disability, forced my development in other areas. I learned to skim-read and was very grateful the day spell check became available. I also developed an ability to focus on long-term projects, because that is what learning to read was for me.

In addition to frustration, the difficulty I had in English class also produced a substantial amount of insecurity. I have struggled with this my entire life. This fed into my love of athletics. Athletics often helped balance a day. If English class had been particularly tough, the day would change for the better when I got to the playground or playfield. There may have been a time or two when I helped my team win. Team members love you when you help them win.

After experiencing some success at the city and county levels of track, I was 13 and I wanted to play football in high school. I started strength training at home with a ramshackle set of weights and a homemade wood bench press in the room next to the garage. There was an old medicine cabinet with a mirror on the floor that leaned at an angle, and I could check my form. After only a short time I noticed bicep growth and the appearance of a vein in my arm, and I was hooked.

At Santa Ana High School, I played football and ran track. I loved these sports. I had been blessed with good genetics, which allowed me to be used by my football coaches in a number of positions.

About the Author

In track, the 330-yard low hurdles event was added when I was a sophomore. My mother suggested I try it. I did and loved it because it was challenging. I had good 440 speed and always helped our mile relay team, but I wasn't fast enough to dominate a 440 dash. The 330 low hurdles was perfect for me and became my main event.

My best friend is still George Jackson. We met on the track team at Santa Ana Community College. He had the classic build of a 400-meter runner: 6' 3" and 185 pounds, with a long fluid stride. I, on the other hand, was not a classic 400 intermediate hurdler. I was 5'8" and 165 pounds. I knew that if I wanted to be competitive I needed to work a little harder than everyone else. I did, and as a sophomore I finished 3rd in the conference finals, which no one expected. Then, I finished 4th in the Southern Sectional Semi Finals with a time of 54.2, missing the finals by one place. That semi final was the fastest I had ever run the 400 hurdles, which was very satisfying, but it also was the finale to my track career. I then attended California State University, Fullerton, (CSUF) which did not have a track team at the time.

SELECTING A CARDIOVASCULAR PROGRAM

About the time I started at CSUF, I started working at Loeschhorn's in Fountain Valley, CA, which would later become "A Snail's Pace." Loeschhorn's was a running specialty shop and 90% of our customers were marathoners. In the years I worked there I learned a great deal about the technical side of running shoes and running. I also learned a great deal about endurance training, endurance athletes, and the problems which resulted from over-training, poor running form, and bad equipment.

Ironically, for those looking to change their lives by starting an exercise program, if your first choice for the cardiovascular portion of your program is going to be running in order to burn a lot of calories, you must also realize that it is the form of exercise most likely to result in injury. With proper guidance you can greatly reduce the risk of injury. Proper running form, good shoes, and a running program which progresses gradually will help you safely start a running program. Visit my website for more information on having your running form evaluated.

The cardiovascular portion of a global fitness program is perhaps the most important because it strengthens the most important muscle in your body: your heart. I have witnessed too many people, including myself, suffer substantial injuries while running. However, I learned from those injuries and I will use this information to help you avoid them. Even if you follow a great running program, your body may not tolerate the pounding that occurs. In that event, you will need to try something else.

I have found cycling to be the most fun cardiovascular exercise when compared to running or swimming. Although it does not burn calories at the same rate as running, it is still a great workout. It's also fun because you are going fast. Unlike running and swimming, when cycling there is some risk of injury due to crashes; however, it is possible to substantially mitigate this risk by riding smart. Another reason I like cycling is because a good bike is a relatively affordable toy. It's healthy to have an object to focus on for a few minutes a week, to make sure it is clean and ready to run smoothly. If that object also contributes to one's fitness, there is no down side.

Swimming is another great cardiovascular exercise. I recommend swimming because it is another form of exercise which rarely causes injury. The other tremendous benefit to swimming is that it is a two-for-one workout. After a good swim you have worked most of the muscles in your entire body. After swimming, in addition to feeling like I just did a great upper-body strength training workout, I know I have just done a great cardiovascular workout too. This makes swimming incredibly efficient, by getting a strength training and cardio workout at the same time.

About the Author

Of course, there is more nomenclature associated with swimming, since you will need to find a pool with hours of operation consistent with when you want to swim. With running and biking, most of us can just head out the front door and start. With swimming, you will need to find a lap pool, pay a small fee, and then use the pool when it's open. So, swimming takes a little more planning, but it's worth it. Also, you don't burn calories quite as fast when swimming as with biking and running, but because it's essentially a two for one workout, again, it's worth it. Also, if you don't have a swimming background, don't expect to be fast or to be able to swim for a long time right away. Swimming fast is highly dependent on form, so you will need to be patient, and you should also plan to get some coaching if you want to get really good. Even if you have poor form, it is still a great workout.

My recommendations of cycling, swimming, and running for cardiovascular exercise are not meant to discount other forms of cardiovascular exercise. They are simply the ones I know best, and which can be engaged in without the need for a class or even workout partners. This means they are the easiest to fit into a tight schedule, like the one I have had my entire life. However, if you have a gym membership and choose to use the cardio equipment to get your heart rate up, that's fine. The key to cardiovascular training is to find something that works, and then gradually increase the duration of exercise from 30 to 60 minutes.

Much of what is in this book I have learned from Bob Forster, world-renowned physical therapist, trainer, and author who has worked with many Olympic champions, world-record holders, and professional athletes. In addition to the pros, Bob has also treated tens of thousand of "regular Joes" like me, so he knows what works. I am living proof. The best part: it is all natural. The supplements I recommend are all natural, and they are exactly what your body needs to maximize the gains made during each workout, through maximizing the recovery process. I have also done extensive additional research and confirmed or enhanced the foundation I learned from Bob. The result is a program based on great fundamentals, not gimmicks or hype.

BAKER TO VEGAS

I am a sprinter by trade. As a sophomore in college I ran the 100 meters in about 11 seconds. I have a lot of fast-twitch muscle fiber, which was great for the positions I played in football. I could change direction and accelerate pretty quickly. At age 32, I began my career with the FBI, and would start training for the office team, which competed in a race called Baker to Vegas. I began running 30 to 40 miles a week, but didn't have any plan.

The Los Angeles office of the FBI has always participated in this race, the largest law enforcement relay in the world, a 120-mile-long race from Baker, California to Las Vegas, Nevada. Each team has 20 runners, so each leg is about six miles. The LA team is usually competitive, and even won the race in 1991. This was a real accomplishment, since there were about 700 Agents in the LA office. This was in contrast to other perennial favorite teams, like the Los Angeles Police Department, Los Angeles County Sheriff's Department, and the California Highway Patrol, which each had from 8,000 to 10,000 officers or deputies from which to field teams.

I had maxed the FBI fitness test at the FBI Academy, so on my arrival at the office in Los Angeles, I was marked for recruitment onto our team. Given my nature, they only had to tell me about the race and the kind of odds we faced, and I was in.

In high school I noticed the fastest pure sprinters all ran on their toes, and as a result had well-developed calves. At that time, to strengthen mine, I began running on my toes at all times. Whether running sprint intervals on the track, or running six miles on a training run, I was on my toes.

It worked. My calves got stronger and I was able to lengthen my stride by pushing off harder. In college, I was able to lengthen my stride so I could run 13 steps between each hurdle. However, it would cause numerous injuries as I trained for and competed in Baker to Vegas some 15 years later, because the calves are meant for use in a sprint stride, not a distance stride.

In my early to mid 30s, my training regimen had no method. I would run four to five times a week, for two or three months before the race, get faster, and then run the qualification course. It was easy.

In the first few years, I ran times among the fastest qualifiers on the team two weeks before the race. I think it was around 1996 or 1997 when I suffered my first calf injury. For the next several years, I would run the same way: train for a few months, run a good qualification time, and then pull a calf muscle two weeks before the race. Each year, I would get physical therapy from Bob and be recovered enough to race. This pattern would turn out to be a blessing in disguise.

The Los Angeles FBI is located in West Los Angeles, very near the UCLA campus. One of the reasons my office won in 1991 was because we had an Olympic-caliber distance runner in the office. As an elite athlete, he had a connection to the trainer for Jackie Joyner Kersey, Robert "Bob" Forster. Bob worked closely with Jackie's coach and husband, Bob Kersey. Bob Forster had a physical therapy facility in nearby Santa Monica: Forster Physical Therapy.

During my first visit, I explained a bit of my athletic background and how I had become injured. I explained that it was very important for me to run the race, which was just a few weeks away. After doing a structural evaluation of me, he paused and told one of his staff to "get him ready to run."

The treatments were the most painful thing I have ever experienced. This was the result of the deep tissue massage from the physical therapy and evidence of how I had misused my calves, causing extensive damage over the years. I also clearly remember during that first evaluation, when Bob began to dig around in my calf to locate the injury, there was not a place on either calf he could touch which did not cause excruciating pain. He was barely pressing on various areas of my calf and I almost came off the table each time. He looked at me and I asked, "Is it supposed to be that painful?" He laughed a little and said, "No." He then told me he was surprised I had been able to train as long and hard as I had with calf muscles which were that tight.

I think it was the third year when Bob recognized the pattern and put me on a treadmill to evaluate my stride. It was the first time he had seen my loping stride. With that stride, my heels never actually struck the ground. He immediately recognized the problem. He told me calf muscles were not designed to do as much work as I was having them do. He explained that calf muscles were meant for sprinting and that it was no wonder I had become injured. He told me I needed to shorten my stride to 180 strides per minute and that such a change could likely resolve my issues. I had heard him, but would not listen to him for several years.

Bob told me, in addition to completely changing my stride I needed to use a program called periodization. He explained that it was a program developed in the Soviet Union in an attempt to demonstrate political and societal superiority through outstanding athletic performance. He said the studies were documented and that the program would help me stay fast, and more importantly, avoid injury. I asked, "Weren't the Soviets well-known to have used performance-enhancing drugs?" He said they were, but the program he recommended did not include the performance-enhancing drugs, just the performance-enhancing workouts.

The last injury I would suffer before adopting the program would occur while racing in Baker to Vegas. I had been given an easier downhill leg and felt pretty good the first couple of miles.

But then I called the follow vehicle up and told them I had just felt a pop in my calf and that I would run until it gave way completely. I told the alternate runner to get ready. I was able to find an alternate foot plant and stride making it possible to hand the baton to the next runner, but I had a nice black and blue patch on the lower part of my calf at the point of the muscle strain.

That year, when I saw Bob after the race for treatment, he pitched me again on changing my stride and that I needed to train using periodization. After years of hearing him talk about this program, I was finally ready to listen. It was 2003 and I was at the brink of athletic disaster. I wasn't ready to stop competing. Adopting the program gave me a new lease on my athletic career.

THE CHANGE THAT BROUGHT ME BACK FROM THE BRINK

Bob worked with me on the treadmill to shorten my stride. He would count each foot plant for 10 seconds and if the count was less than 30, I had to shorten my stride. The goal was to have 30 foot plants in 10 seconds. You multiply 30 by six to get to the goal of 180. By the time I was able to run the 180 strides per minute, it felt like my strides were half the length of my "normal" stride. On faith, I started using the new stride and the long-range results have exceeded my expectations.

The increase in cadence allowed my foot to land below my body's center of gravity, which then allowed for a midfoot strike rather than a forefoot strike. This meant my calves were doing much less work and the big pusher muscles, the quadriceps and glutes, were taking up a majority of the work. The first year, I wasn't quite as fast as I had been several years before, but I made it to the race without injury, which was the first victory.

We also talked about my training program for running and found another problem. I didn't really have a program or system as a guide. I just ran whatever felt right on a given day, with no regard for recovery.

In college, I did strength training a couple of nights a week in the same gym as my brother, who was a nationally ranked 242-pound power lifter. Power lifting involves three lifts: bench press, squat, and deadlift. This was the early '80s, so I adopted a strength-training program similar to my brother's bench press routine, but with much less weight. After college, I did not do any strength training for my legs. I mistakenly believed I did not need to do strength training for my legs, and that running was enough. I was wrong.

For the next 20 years I would do the same bench press routine, which involved one light and one heavy bench day each week. My heavy bench days were Fridays, and involved multiple repetitions with 275 pounds and more. This would lead to a shoulder injury, which would require surgery.

In 2002, I noticed a soreness deep inside my left shoulder when I did bench press and pull-ups. Over several months the pain became more pronounced. I had worked "through" many injuries over the years and I presumed I would be able to work through this one too. At one point, I rested my shoulder and stopped doing bench press and pull-ups for a while, and it got a little better. But when I started doing them again, I was left with a steady dull pain.

I called Bob and asked his opinion. He referred me to an orthopedic surgeon, Dr. Thomas Knapp. Dr. Knapp identified the injury as an issue with the labrum and recommended physical therapy, since the extent of the injury could not be easily determined. For six months I underwent physical therapy and almost all of the pain in the shoulder went away and my shoulder became stronger. Between the rest, deep tissue massages, electro stimulation, and light and very controlled strength training during physical therapy, my shoulder greatly improved.

Then, one afternoon my youngest daughter, who was three at

the time, bumped my arm. It was really nothing more than a slight nudge, but the angle of my arm was just so, and it caused a shooting pain in my shoulder. Clearly, although my shoulder had become much stronger, the injury was not any better. We had given it a great try by using physical therapy, the least invasive methodology, to try to resolve the injury without surgery. However, after six months of physical therapy, the time for surgery had arrived. The shoulder issue coincided with my history of leg injuries. What was happening to me? With the multiple issues, I was ready for the changes I would need to make, and I was lucky to already have a relationship with someone I trusted, and who also had the deep body of knowledge I would need.

After the shoulder surgery, Bob assigned physical therapist Gray O'Brien to treat me. He quickly and correctly identified my type-"A" personality. He continually reinforced the idea that, if I was going to recover quickly and completely from this injury and successful surgery, I would be required to follow his strength training and stretching protocol to the letter. This would require patience. At 42, this notion ran counter to my instincts and previous practices, but he said it often enough that I listened. In fact, Gray admitted at the end of the PT that at the beginning of treatment he believed I would not make it through all eight weeks of PT as a result of my nature. We laughed.

At the end of the two months, my shoulder was healed and strong enough to curtail PT. Grey implored me to continue using all of the shoulder exercises he had shown me. He also recommended using periodization for all of my strength training. I did. After 10 years, I am literally in the best shape of my life.

Another benefit of my shoulder PT was that it also healed a problem I'd had for more than a decade with my other shoulder. The bicep tendon in my right shoulder had given me problems when throwing a ball, and on occasion when bench pressing. Since I had followed the stretching and strength-training protocols for both shoulders during PT, the problem with the bicep tendon in the right shoulder also resolved. Through discipline and great PT, we had resolved a problem we weren't even addressing. This has happened with several other athletes I have trained using this program.

Becoming a Coach

To qualify for the Los Angeles FBI Office's Open team you must try out. We have a 5.7 mile course nearby, and if your time is fast enough, you can win a spot on the team. After I began using the program, my qualifying times got a little faster. I also began using a heart rate monitor (HRM), which allowed me to train and race to my full potential, by controlling my early exertion so I would have something left at the end. In endurance races, the goal is to run "negative splits." A negative split means the miles at the end of the race are faster than those at the beginning. Prior to using a HRM, because of adrenaline, I have always started too fast and would run the first mile much faster than I should have. The result was that I would often struggle all the way to the finish line, and experience far more discomfort than necessary. This practice made trying out and racing a very painful experience.

When I started using the HRM, coupled with testing which told me my various pulse ranges, I started running smarter. I replaced instinct and adrenaline with good data and patience, and started getting faster.

From that point, at the start of a tryout run, which would include many younger agents, these younger agents would take off like they were shot from cannons. Fighting my "chase" instinct and having faith in the program, I let them go, while I would stay in my pulse range. There is a steep hill in the middle of the course and that is where I would start to catch many of the guys who had taken off so fast to start. I would then start picking the rest of them off, one by one. By the end of a tryout I was often among the fastest. After the tryouts, a number of the younger agents asked me what I was doing to be strong at the end of the run. I told them about the program.

After a few years I found myself coaching a number of people in the office, including quite a few female agents who would run on the women's team. Eventually, I was asked to write the program down, and did. In every case, when the program was followed closely, the athletes have gotten faster, without injury.

One of the most dramatic improvements I have seen was a female agent I coached who wanted to run on the Women's' Baker to Vegas team. She did not have a running or even athletic background, but she wanted to try to make the team. She had also suffered from chronic shin splints and was running between 9 and 10 minute miles for a 10K at the time I started working with her. In her third year of using the program, she ran sub-7 minute miles on the track and did not have shin splints. I remember that day on the track when she broke the 7-minute barrier. She was surprised and very excited. However, initially, she thought she had made a mistake in her timing. Then, when she ran another mile in under 7 minutes, she knew it was real.

Since then, many of the athletes I have coached have had similar experiences. My own wife asked me to coach her. She was running 9 plus- minute miles. Then, after a couple of years, she ran under 8 minute miles during a couple of track workouts. What made this especially significant was that she was coming back from having had a hysterectomy when she broke the 8-minute barrier for the first time. She was in very good shape before the surgery, since she knew it would help speed her recovery. Then, only a few months after starting to train again, she went with me to the track. The day she broke the 8-minute barrier, she too was surprised and ecstatic.

3. Periodization or Something Else

THE OVERARCHING PRINCIPLE OF PERIODIZATION IS: GRADUAL smart improvement. This runs counter to what many people want: very fast results with little effort or discipline. There are many exercise and diet programs that may achieve relatively quick results; however, in many cases the results can be quickly lost because the intensity is not sustainable. They require only a short commitment. They may create some improvement in specific fitness or weight loss, but they often result in what I call "stock market" fitness. In such programs, you invest a great deal of effort over a short period of time, which may improve your fitness to a degree, but it will do virtually nothing for your health. It is possible in some cases to see dramatic improvement, but because these programs are not designed with long-term fitness or health in mind, when the workout or diet regimen ends, you end up losing all the gains you made, and more.

Super-intense programs are not sustainable, and in many cases they do little to improve your cardiovascular system. In most cases, traditional fitness regimens like swimming, biking, or running are far superior when compared to quick workout gimmicks. Also, because of the burnout often associated with super-high intensity programs and very restrictive diets, in many cases, when people stop using one of these programs they completely stop working out and usually gain back any weight they have lost, plus additional weight. The idea that you can make meaningful, substantial, and lasting fitness or health gains in a very short period of time is simply not true. Real fitness and health don't involve hype and gimmicks; they involve the use over time of great fundamentals.

Periodization or Something Else

To make meaningful, substantial, safe, and lasting health and fitness gains, it will take some time. The truth is that you need to find about an hour a day to improve or maintain a higher level of health and fitness. I should also say that it is possible to see improvements in a number of areas in just a few weeks; however, substantial gains will take months and years to achieve. But, they are gains you will have for the rest of your life. You must make the commitment to yourself, to take good care of yourself, now and for the rest of your life.

Periodization

Periodization is literally about training smarter, not harder. That's not to say this program does not contain workouts in which you will exert greatly -- it does. However, because of the scientific nature of the program, you will gradually work up to the high-intensity workouts, so they will be part of a relatively easy and natural progression.

Periodization has three phases: base, building, and peak. Also, in periodization, volume and intensity have an inverse relationship. That is to say, as intensity increases, volume decreases. As a result, in base phase there is higher volume, but at a lower intensity, while in peak phase the volume will be reduced while the intensity will be increased. Also, the body adapts quickly to any specific exertion, so, after eight weeks in one phase, you move to the next. The changes in exertion at these intervals have been proven the most effective at causing the body to adapt by creating stronger muscles and naturally stimulating the release of beneficial hormones, including testosterone. Periodization is an effective training method for cardiovascular exercise and strength training.

Most athletes I have coached find the low-intensity base phase to be the most difficult part of the program, from a mental rather than physical standpoint. They have a hard time believing and accepting that by running at a slower pace, they can get faster.

This program is counterintuitive. Most of us don't understand how the body gets stronger. The old-school belief regarding distance running was that you needed to run hard every day, or at least five or six days a week. Although widely believed, this was wrong and usually led to injury or burnout, or both. That's because your body needs time to recover. Studies show the specific muscles used during exercise need recovery time to maximize hormone stimulation and increase muscle mass.

Periodization uses the body's natural ability to adapt to get stronger and faster, without injury. The reason people who run every day get injured is because they never let their bodies recover. As you will see, recovery is perhaps the most important part of periodization, and recovery is built into every week, month, and year of training.

Since running requires the most recovery between workouts, I will use it to illustrate. Studies show that, following a run workout, you need about 48 hours of recovery before you should run again. This means only three runs a week are possible. Additionally, studies show that by increasing the workout load gradually, each week for three weeks, and then reducing the volume by 40 % during the fourth week, you will actually be stronger during the fifth week. That's because, during the recovery week the body has a chance to completely heal from the three prior weeks' workouts. This is true for cardiovascular and strength training.

This is the result of the body's natural ability to adapt. When you increase the load gradually, you avoid severely shocking the body, allowing it to adapt instead of breaking down. Later in this book we will discuss injury identification and prevention, so, should you be heading to a possible injury, you will know what it is and what to do about it.

Periodization is good for everyone, whether you have an athletic background or not. In some cases, not having an athletic background could be beneficial. I have coached many runners who did not have athletic backgrounds. In most of those cases, their bodies were "fresh," meaning they did not have pre-existing injuries. Coming from non-athletic backgrounds, they had never pressed themselves earlier in life, so they had no idea what their genetic potential was. For many of these "non-athletes," their workouts to that point in their lives had been unguided and had no structure or method. Then, after consistently training the right way, they obtained the most dramatic improvement of anyone I have coached.

My mother is a prime example of such an athlete. She grew up on a farm in Minnesota. At that time, they did not have organized sports for girls. She was very active on the farm, not just with chores, but in playing sports against her little brother and other boys. She was always faster than the boys.

Not having played organized sports actually turned out to be a benefit for her later in life. After my father passed away in 2003 following a valiant battle with cancer, God rest his soul, one of the things my mom did to help deal with the loss was to start working out. She joined a gym, hired a personal trainer, and started working out two hours a day three times a week.

Even though she was in her 70s, she saw substantial improvement and the trainers gradually and regularly increased the weights she used. They also increased the duration of her cardio training. A couple of years ago she trimmed down by losing some fat. That's not to say she was fat. She was not. However, as happens with many of us, a little fat crept on during her life and she had probably 20 pounds she could afford to lose. As her fitness improved and her muscle mass increased her body mass changed, naturally. She lost the fat without even trying and the muscle she put on, because it is heavier than fat, meant she looked totally ripped but had not lost any weight.

For those like myself with an athletic background, a lot of unlearning will be necessary. The workout methods we used in high school and college were not the results of scientific studies. They were born of informal studies, at best. These routines often did help young athletes perform better, but only because youthful bodies can tolerate abuse better than older bodies. This tolerance of abuse often delayed the appearance of injuries for years. Ironically, convincing older athletes to use periodization can be difficult. I offer my initial resistance as an example.

I have seen many athletes train with injuries for years and, as a result of their ability to tolerate pain, they could continue to train, but by doing so they made the injury more severe with each workout. In some cases, they trained until the injury was so severe they could not continue. When this happens, the injury is sometimes so severe it is not possible to effectively treat it, bringing an end to an athletic career. It doesn't have to be that way. I have convinced many mature athletes with long-term injuries to seek treatment, and when they have, the injuries have resolved, allowing them to resume their athletic careers. So, if you have an injury and are thinking of starting this program, resolve the injury first, and then begin anew.

GETTING IN THE ZONE

To maximize the benefit of this program, you will need to know your heart rate ranges or zones. If you have been training with a HRM but have not been tested to get your aerobic and anaerobic pulse thresholds, you have not been using your HRM to full benefit. There are many fine heart rate monitors available today, which start at about $100. Other HRMs can run as much as $500 and tell you all sorts of information you probably don't need to know, as too much data or looking at the wrong data can be frustrating and overwhelming. When running or biking, all I need to know is my pulse. If I am above my targeted rate I slow down, and if I am below my targeted rate I speed up so I am in the pulse range required for that workout.

When I started using this program I bought the most basic model

HRM, for around $60. It displayed either the pulse rate or the time of day, but not both at the same time. During the base and building phases this was fine because the only thing I needed to know during those workouts was how fast my heart was beating in order to stay in my targeted heart rate zone. If I was not in my zone, I would adjust my pace to raise or lower my heart rate so I was. However, during the peak phase I needed to wear another sport watch with a stopwatch so I could get split times during the track workouts. While wearing two watches worked, I eventually graduated to a newer version HRM, which displayed HR and the stopwatch function at the same time.

There are a lot of HRMs which tell you a lot of other information that you may want to know, but you don't really need to know, like your pace per mile. This can be distracting and restrict your overall progress because a lot of people like to "chase the pace." That is to say, they like running a faster pace because they feel better about running a 7:15 pace rather than a 7:30 pace per mile.

A word of advice: chase pulse and not pace, and let the speed take care of itself. It will come. However, you will need to be patient and let the program work by letting your body adapt. What you will find is that every time you get to your peak phase and time yourself on the track, your times will be a little faster than at the same time during the previous cycle.

So, for anyone using a HRM, the pulse is the most important information on the display. You will have to learn to trust the program and follow your pulse, not chase your pace. To trust the program, you need to know more about what it does.

The Phases

Each phase or "period" of periodization is eight weeks and each phase helps your body develop in specific ways. The phases are eight weeks, because the studies show, after eight weeks your body's ability to adapt has been maximized, and you need to change the stimulus to create additional adaptation. By increasing the load gradually, over time the body changes to accommodate the additional workload while also greatly reducing the risk of injury.

Just as important as increasing the load gradually is recovery. Within the eight-week phases, there will be two so-called "recovery" weeks. During the first three weeks you will add volume each week, and in the fourth week, reduce the volume by 40 to 50%. These recovery weeks are necessary as a result of micro-tears that occur to muscle fibers during exercise. These micro-tears are completely normal, and when volume and intensity are increased properly, they cause the body to increase muscle fiber as part of adaptation. Some recovery occurs during the days between workouts, but complete recovery occurs during these recovery weeks, resulting in noticeable increases in fitness.

By gradually increasing volume or intensity you add stress to your skeleton-muscular and or cardiovascular systems, which causes adaptation. When you add substantial volume or intensity the result is often injury, because you have exceeded your body's ability to adapt. When you increase the physical stress through exercise several things happen. You cause micro-tears in muscle fibers, which causes mild inflammation in various tendons and ligaments. However, if the exercise is at the right volume and intensity, the body will increase muscle fiber, which triggers tendons and ligaments to get thicker and stronger.

When we talk about micro-tears in the muscle fibers, we are talking about extremely small damage caused to the muscle fiber, hence the term "micro-tears." This is the reason you should not run two days in a row. By putting a day of rest in between runs, you let the micro-tears and inflammation resolve to a degree. This is why gradual progress is so important, so you don't create more physiological stress than your body can handle, which usually results in injuries.

This program will change your body, first internally, which increases efficiency and durability. This usually leads to external changes you can see, like a reduction in body fat and improved muscular definition. This is due in part to the production of hormones. The recovery periods promote the natural enhancement of the body's ability to produce hormones, which then maximizes adaptation, triggering substantial increases in strength and speed.

BASE PHASE

For most cardiovascular training, you must go slow to go fast. For strength training, you must lift light weights to get stronger. Going slow or lifting lighter weights is the toughest concept in this program, but you must trust the program and let it work. By using base-phase training you will literally make yourself a better-functioning machine.

One of the reasons base phase is so difficult is because, in most cases, the pace you will run or ride in order to stay in the appropriate heart rate range will be much slower than you can run or ride. The same is true with strength training. I have coached some runners who, after getting their heart rate "zones" through testing, have experienced significant frustration. When they started the program, in order to stay in their base heart rate range, they were running so slowly they were almost walking. For those who were disciplined enought to trust and follow the program, they were met with very positive results.

From my days working at Loeschhorn's until today, I have heard hundreds if not thousands of stories of people starting run programs the wrong way, with too much volume and intensity too early. They run two miles the first day and feel great so they run three miles the next time they run, and keep adding another mile every run, and they feel great. But then after about two weeks, various joints and muscles start to get really sore as they start to break down. As discussed above, this is the result of not allowing the body to recover and heal completely. By not allowing the body to heal, the micro-tears and inflammation accumulate and then muscles get tight, which starts to cause biomechanical issues. Add these problems together, and injuries usually follow.

To avoid this, you must start and progress gradually, as you will see in the "Starting From '0' Mileage" protocol detailed later. I have used this protocol several times myself and know many others who have used it, with great success.

You will need to find a way to be patient and let the base phase improve your fitness in unseen ways. Running at a lower pulse range prevents excessive strain on muscles and also helps to make tendons and ligaments stronger. Improved tendon and ligament strength is essential to tolerate the increased intensity you will place on the system later during the building and peak phases. Remember, we are going to build muscular strength gradually, so we need to do the same with tendons and ligaments. Muscles grow faster than tendons and ligaments, so a gradual increase in strength training and cardiovascular volume will allow everything to stay in balance. This is an important part of the program and is a major reason this program helps prevent injury. Additionally, when tendons, ligaments, and muscles get stronger, the increased muscular strength triggers adaptation in the bones to which they are attached, resulting in increased bone density.

The base phase also makes your cardiovascular system more efficient by enhancing capillary development. Capillaries are the tiny blood vessels that deliver fuel to and remove waste products from muscles. Muscles need fuel, which is used to cause contractions. While contracting, muscles produce waste products that need to be taken away. These waste products pass through capillaries and into the blood stream for removal. When you have better capillary development, you increase your capacity to exercise at a higher rate and

Periodization or Something Else

for a longer period of time because your body is able to exchange fuel and waste at a greater capacity and with greater efficiency.

Lastly, and perhaps the best reason for following the base phase of the program is that you burn mostly fat as a fuel source in this phase. Bob calls it "being a better butter burner." The human body has several sources of fuel, and the percentage of fuel used from each system is determined by the intensity of exertion. At lower exertion rates, fat is the primary fuel source, while at higher exertion rates the primary fuel shifts to mostly carbohydrates.

Studies show that the human body can store from 30 to 90 minutes of carbohydrates, which can be used for fuel during exercise. These same studies show that the human body has a much higher amount of fuel stored as fat. When you become a "better butter burner," you begin to change your body composition by losing stored fat, which makes you lighter. As is said in car racing, lighter is faster. But you have to train your body to use fat, which is why the first two months of the program requires you to train in your base pulse range.

Building Phase

The building phase is the transitional phase. It is the phase that prepares your body to eventually endure the peak-phase intensity. During the base phase you have improved tendon and ligament strength, muscular endurance, bone density, capillary development, and your body's ability to burn fat. These structural improvements will result in better power, speed, and endurance in the peak phase. However, it is too much strain on your body to go right from the rates of exertion in base phase to those in peak phase, and so we move to the building phase.

I always feel liberated when I go from base to building phase. Instead of having to continually check my pulse and then slow down my pace in order to bring my pulse down into my base phase range,

I get to run and ride more freely. I still check the pulse regularly to ensure I am "in range." Also, during the building phase, the longer weekend training sessions are still in the base-pulse range. That's to keep your body familiar with burning fat as a fuel source, while still keeping your volume high but at a lower intensity, to help reduce the risk of injury.

Peak Phase

After two months of training long and slow in the base phase, and then two months at an intermediate pace during the building phase, it is time to start getting really strong and fast. For running and cycling, peak phase involves interval work and hills at or near your anaerobic threshold (AT). AT is associated with a high level of exertion and the specific heart rate at which you begin to go into oxygen debt and start to produce very high levels of lactic acid. The amount of lactic acid produced at or above your AT is more than your body can clear for a long time. You can continue to function at or above your AT, but only for short periods of time. With proper training and the use of a HRM, you can change your AT so you can exert at a higher level for a longer period of time, which is the purpose of the peak phase.

However, during peak-phase training, you will still do longer weekend workouts, but they will be in base-pulse range. These longer and lower-intensity workouts keep the body familiar with burning fat while also keeping intensity and the risk of injury low, while keeping the volume high.

The best way to increase the intensity during the peak phase involves interval training, working in pulse ranges which are at or near your AT. The best way to ensure you are in the right pulse range is to use a HRM and to know your pulse ranges from a test which measures your Maximum Oxygen uptake Volume (VO2 Max) or one which measures the amount of lactic acid your body produces, known as the Blood Lactate Test (BLT). These are explained in greater detail later.

It is possible to get a rough idea of your AT for running by following the protocol below, and it still requires the use of a HRM. Test yourself this way only after completing the base and building phases first. On a 400-meter track, run two laps at a fast pace and pay attention to your breathing. After two laps, if you are running fast enough, your breathing will change from breathing hard, which is sustainable, to hyperventilation, which is not sustainable. The difference between breathing hard and hyperventilation is different for everyone, so there is not a set rate of "breaths per minute" I can give you to differentiate between the two. So, when you reach a rate of breathing you feel you cannot sustain, slow your pace slightly until you are no longer hyperventilating, and are just breathing really hard. After a few seconds, look at your HRM, and that will be pretty close to your AT. To reiterate, this is a non-scientific way to determine an approximate AT. The best way to determine your AT, and other important pulse ranges, is to get a VO2 test or a BLT. Check my website for more information.

By design, we have our different fuel sources, which have benefited our development as a species. If we think about ourselves and how we were originally designed as predators, if we were following prey at a walking or jogging pace, waiting for the prey to tire, we could do this for a long time because we would be in an aerobic state. With a low pulse, we would burn mostly fat as an energy source. When the prey grew tired, we would shift gears to carefully stalk the prey so we could get close enough to pounce or attack. When sprinting for a short distance to exploit the element of surprise and quickly close the final few meters, we would shift to an anaerobic state and use mostly fast burning carbohydrates for fuel. In the sprint, we would extend our stride, run on our toes, and be able to sustain this exertion for only a short time.

During the peak phase we will work on increasing the load on the muscles to make them stronger, and we will also hold these exertion rates for long enough to enhance the cardiovascular system to deliver fuel and remove waste from the muscles with greater efficiency. In doing so, we will improve our cardiovascular system and begin to change our AT.

Through hill and interval training we will improve your range of motion, muscular strength, and cardiovascular system, which will result in an increase in sustainable speed.

In peak-phase running workouts, we will not try to increase our speed by doing wind-sprints, 400-meter or 800-meter intervals. Though many high school and college athletes use these distances to increase leg speed, they carry a high risk of injury for "mature" athletes. Such distances are also too short to create any real benefit for your cardiovascular system.

For running, I use and recommend 1-mile intervals on a track. The reason I recommend intervals of 1 mile is because for individuals with a good cardiovascular base, it should take about 800 meters -- or two laps around a track -- just to get to your AT. This means if you were running an interval of 800 meters you would stop running just as you reached the desired heart rate. Only by running for a period after that do you force the body to become more efficient at delivering fuel to and removing waste products from muscles.

The same principle is applied when running or riding hills, which is why it will be important to find longer hills to climb. If it takes only a couple of minutes to reach the top of a hill, you won't be at or near your AT for long enough to cause meaningful cardiovascular adaptation. You will derive some muscular benefit on such hills, but to maximize your body's ability to adapt you will need to find hills which take five to 10 minutes or more to climb.

4. Mechanics of Running

RUNNING IS DANGEROUS. IT IS KNOWN TO CAUSE THE MOST INJUries of the three cardiovascular exercises described in this book. However, improper training and bad form or both cause most of these injuries, which means they are preventable. It is also true that running burns the most calories of these exercises, giving it the most risk with the most potential reward. Like most of life, running is about managing risk. With a proper training schedule, as detailed below, coupled with proper running form, running can be one of the most efficient forms of exercise to improve or maintain high levels of fitness and health.

Although I go into great detail about proper running form, you may still need more guidance than I can provide in this book to overcome specific issues. In that case, I recommend getting a "run gait analysis" from a qualified expert. I have links on my website to some of the foremost experts in the field. With a smart phone, treadmill, and a friend to video record you, you can e-mail the video for a complete run gait analysis.

I highly recommend a run gait analysis for almost everyone who plans to take up running. Very few people have naturally perfect running form, and as I watch people run on the street every day, I see that most of them have significant issues, which can easily lead to injury. Just as easily, these issues can be corrected, with proper guidance. The time, effort, and money invested to make sure you are on the right track will be well spent, given the reduction in the risk of injury which will follow.

For distance running, a natural foot plant involves a light strike on the outside of the heel or midfoot. As weight transfers forward to the ball of the foot the "toe off" should be neutral. If your heel rolls quickly to the inside following the heel strike before rolling to the forefoot, you have a condition called pronation. This can cause knee and other issues, and in most cases can be corrected. If you pronate, go to a good running store that has a treadmill with cameras. They should be able to see your foot pronate and then put you in a shoe that can correct the movement. Running shoe stores with a treadmill camera generally have the expertise to solve the problem with the right shoe, or they can recommend a good podiatrist or physical therapist who can provide custom orthotics.

Proper body position when running longer distances means your torso is neutral, straight up and down, or you have a very slight forward lean. The foot should land almost directly under the torso. When viewed from the front or rear, ankles, knees, and hips should be in the same plane. If after you start running you feel pain in your knees, ankles, or hips, which lasts from one workout to the next, have a sports medicine doctor, a good physical therapist, or a podiatrist evaluate you.

A lot of people "shuffle run." This means their feet and knees stay low to the ground. This is a very inefficient and slow way to run. When viewed from the side, heels and knees should be relatively high. By having high heels, which means the lower leg is roughly parallel to the ground at its highest point, less effort is required to rotate at the hip to bring the knee forward and up. To test this, stand next to a chair with one hand on the chair and swing the outside leg forward and back, moving only at the hip. Keep your leg straight while you swing it. Then, while still swinging your leg back and forth, bend your leg at the knee so your lower leg is parallel to the ground, and feel how much easier and faster your leg swings. That's the result of having shortened the lever -- your leg, in this case -- which was accomplished by bringing your lower leg closer to your body. Shortening your lever represents a mechanical improvement, meaning it takes less energy to move the leg back and forth. There is an aerodynamic benefit as well. By raising your knees, you decrease aerodynamic "drag" by reducing the surface area of your leg, which must push through the air. This reduction in drag means it will take less energy to move forward and will also likely produce an increase in speed.

In proper distance running form, your torso should remain quiet. That is to say, your torso should not move from side to side and should not rotate much. If you think of each hip and shoulder as being corners of a table, the table should remain square to the direction you are running, with only a slight rotation of the hips. This promotes the best mechanical position for your muscles used for running. You will have very powerful muscles like quads, glutes, and hamstrings pulling against your pelvis and lower back. The hip flexor attaches at the top of your thigh bone and connects to your lower spine. You will also have the torque of your arm swing trying to rotate your shoulders, and all of this counter-rotation means you will need a strong core to make it all work. Again, when I talk about core strength I am talking about strong abs, lower back and oblique muscles. You will see how to strengthen these in the strength training section.

Back to your torso as a table top: the idea is to keep the table square to your direction of travel, with the legs moving back and forth; with ankles, knees, and hips all in line, and arms swinging back and forth in a straight line, without coming across your body or flaring away from the sides of your torso. The best way to visualize proper arm swing is to think about ears and pockets. In the forward position, your hand should be in a position to touch your earlobe on that side. You won't actually touch your ear, but it must be in line to do so. When your hand is back it should be in position to touch a front pocket on that side. Hands coming across your body wastes energy because they are moving laterally. Running is about moving forward, not sideways. So, any part of your body that moves sideways slows you down and wastes energy. When trying to fix your arm swing, think about "ears and pockets." Arms should be bent at the elbow at about a 90-degree angle. Just as the direction of arm-swing is important, so is the amount of travel your upper arm has moving forward and to the rear. In efficient distance running, most of the arm swing will be to the rear of your torso in order to balance your leg travel, most of which should also happen behind the midpoint of your torso. That is to say, your upper arms should swing much farther to the rear than to the front of your torso.

Hands should be relaxed, not straight as a board or clenched in a fist. I have heard proper hand position described as being relaxed enough to hold a potato chip. To find this position, stand up and let your arms and hands relax. The natural position your hands are in at that time is very close to the position they should be in when running.

Shoulders need to be relaxed, which means low. A lot of untrained runners tend to hold their shoulders very high, or hunched. This wastes energy and binds the upper body. Low and loose shoulders allow everything else in a running stride to function better. When starting a running program, think about shoulders occasionally and make sure they are low and loose.

Your cadence should be 180 strides per minute. When converting to this stride many years ago I was on the treadmill and had to keep shortening my stride until it felt like I was taking baby steps. It took a few weeks to get used to it, but now it feels natural. The benefit of taking 180 strides per minute is that it promotes a foot strike below your torso with a light heel strike, and also engages the big "pusher" muscles, the quads and glutes. By shortening your stride you increase the number of strides needed to cover the same distance, but you also decrease the load placed on those muscles for each stride. Studies show that, even though you are taking a great number of strides, the decreased load per stride is the most efficient for running long distances.

MECHANICS OF RUNNING

To test your cadence, run on a treadmill and count the number of foot strikes you have in 10 seconds. If you have 30, your cadence is 180. However, most people will have many fewer strides. Just like I did, you will need to shorten your stride to take more steps until you count to 30 just as the clock gets to 10 seconds.

ILLUSTRATION OF: MECHANICS OF RUNNING

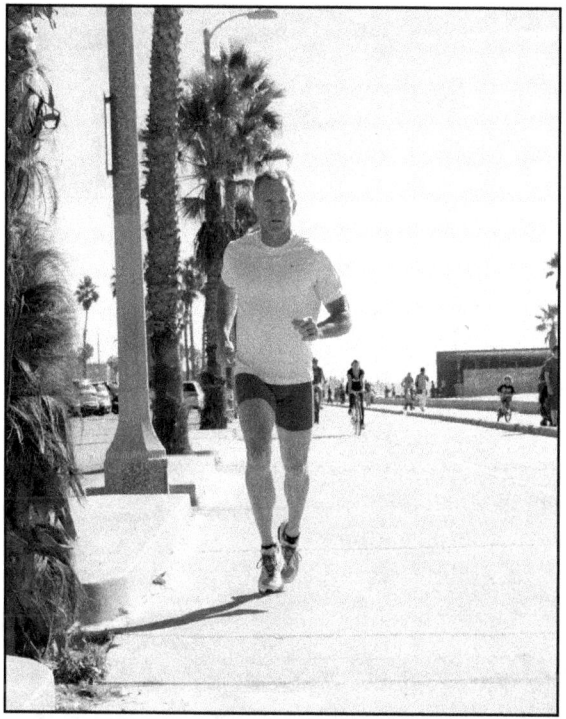

Photos by: Felicity Murphy

In this front view my shoulders are pretty square and there is a slight rotation in my hips. My arms are on a plane from my pocket to my ear. Although I have slightly bowed lower legs, my hips, knees, and ankles still line up pretty well.

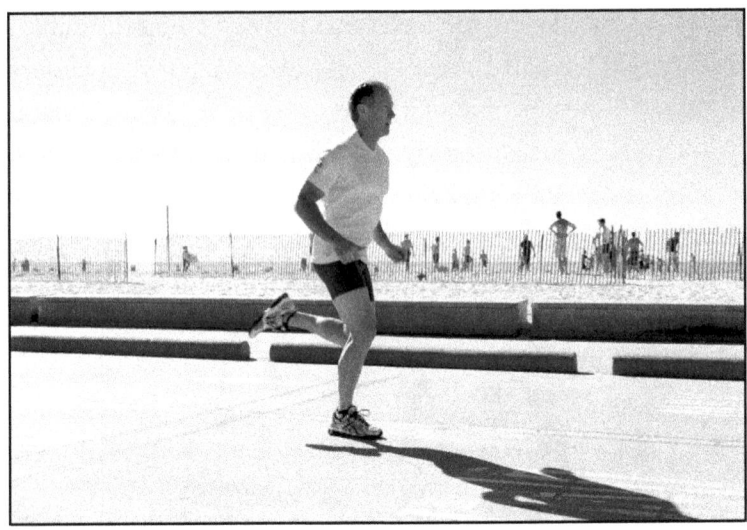

This shows a high heel in the transition phase of my stride. The arm nearest the camera is as far back as it will go.

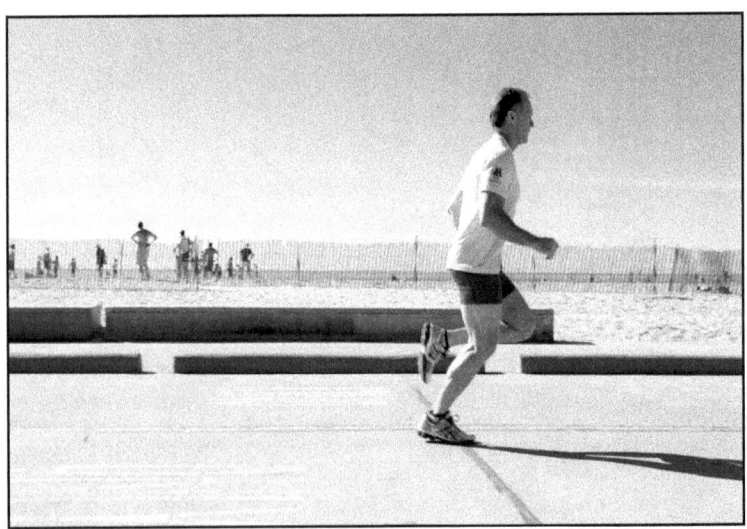

The knee is high during the drive phase of my stride and my elbow angle is a constant 90 degrees.

Mechanics of Running

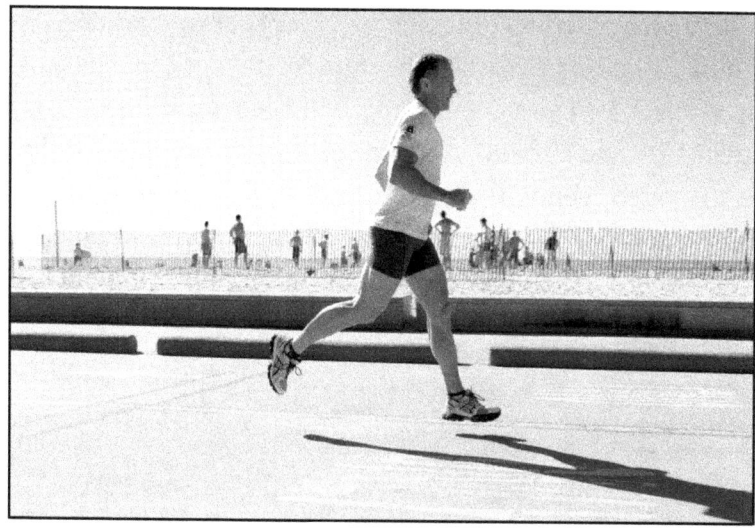

My lower leg is in front of my torso and my arm is as far forward as it will go.

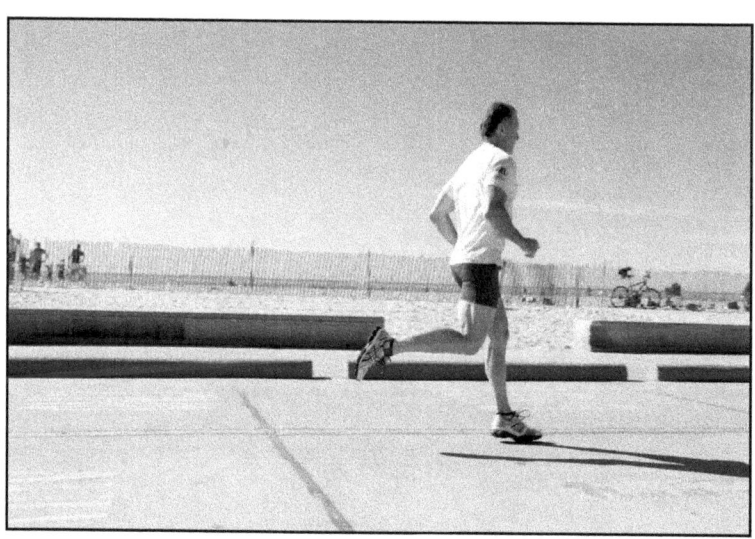

Here I am just making contact. It is a pretty neutral contact, with a slight tip down of my forefoot and my foot is very close to underneath my torso.

If following the directions above doesn't get your stride to where you think it should be, it might be time for a video gait analysis. Go to my website for more details. You will need a smartphone, access to a treadmill, and a friend. After following the directions on how to shoot the video, you will e-mail it to one of the sites. A stride mechanics expert will evaluate your stride and provide detailed feedback in a return e-mail on how you can make improvements.

5. Mechanics of Cycling

Although I am relatively new to cycling, as a result of having trained for a couple of years for triathlons, I have learned that the most important thing about proper mechanics when cycling is having the right size bike. What you plan to do with the bike becomes the next most important thing. If you plan to ride trails in your local hills and mountains, then the answer is simple: you need a mountain bike. However, if you want to start by riding a bike on the road, the answer to the question of which bike will be right for you involves several factors.

If you have lower back flexibility issues, you may want to consider a hybrid road bike, which will put you in a more upright position. If flexibility is not an issue, you may want to consider a road bike. If you think you might want to train for and compete in triathlons and you can afford only one bike, you may want to consider what's called a time trial or "TT" bike. Keep in mind though, that TT bikes are generally preferred for triathlons because they put you in a more aerodynamic position. However, this position is also considered by many to be less comfortable than the more upright position of a standard road bike.

Although which bike you buy is important, getting the right size is even more so. If you don't get the right size, it will not be possible to fit you to the bike correctly, which will negatively affect how comfortable you are on the bike as well as how powerful and efficient you will be. To make sure you get the right size bike, go to a high-end bike shop and get evaluated. Some shops will do this for free, hoping you will buy a bike from them; others will charge a small fee if you don't buy from them. Once you have that information, you will need to buy the bike and then get a proper fit.

Once you are on the right bike and in the right position, it's time to maximize your pedal stroke. Watts are used to measure the power output in a pedal stroke. Using more of the correct muscles when pedaling a bike will result in the production of more watts. Proper riding form coupled with the use of periodization will result in an increase in watt production over time by increasing the muscle mass used to create power.

A proper pedal stroke is not just pushing down hard on the pedals. This is sometimes referred to as "mashing" the pedals. Like running, pedaling efficiently means pedaling at a certain rate per minute, called cadence. Optimal cadence for most riders is between 85 and 95. I recommend you buy a bike computer that measures cadence, speed, and distance. There are a lot of bike computers that measure many other parameters. Just like in running, it's not about how much data you collect and use, it's more about collecting and using the right data points, or suffering the fate of being overwhelmed by data.

A cadence of around 90 is faster than most people naturally ride. However, by riding at a tempo that is a little higher, you reduce the energy needed to turn each pedal stroke. Even though you will have more pedal strokes to cover a given distance, the energy needed to generate each pedal stroke will be less.

If this sounds similar to the principles of the most efficient running stride, it is. Bike cadence is based on one foot completing a revolution, while running cadence is measured with each foot strike. This means the optimal cadence for running, 180 foot strikes per minute, and for cycling, 90 complete revolutions of one foot per minute, are the same, since if you count the revolutions of each foot, 90 X 2 = 180.

Although riding a bike is relatively simple, maximizing your power output for each pedal stroke involves more than meets the eye. Good cyclists don't just push down on the pedal. Good cyclists usually apply some pressure to the pedal in every part of the stroke. That is to say, when the pedal is near the bottom of the stroke, they pull back using their hamstrings and as the pedal rises they pull up with their hip flexor. To complete a pedal stroke, as the pedal starts to move forward they push the pedal forward using their quads. To be clear, they are not pulling or pushing as hard as they can in every phase of a pedal stroke. They save that for hard climbs or sprints. However, during most riding they are usually applying at least some pressure to each part of the stroke, as opposed to just pushing down on the pedal, which uses mostly glutes and quads.

To develop a more complete pedal stroke, you can do several exercises. But before we get to the exercises, I recommend you use what are called clipless pedals. These are the types of pedals which have a cleat which attaches to your shoe, which then allows the shoe to attach to the pedal. Such pedals help to transfer more power into the bike and to the road, which helps you go faster.

I will admit I have always been a little confused by the term "clipless" pedals, because when I use them they actually make a clicking noise as I secure my shoes to pedals. If I may digress, the term clipless pedal comes from the development of the type of pedal most cyclists use now, which was different from how good cyclists used to secure their feet to their pedals.

The old system used what they called toe clips. This system used a metal fitting which was attached to the front of a conventional pedal and curved over the toe of the shoe and had a piece of leather which encircled the shoe and pedal just forward of the arch. The leather strap could then be pulled tight using a buckle or spring tension system, securely attaching the rider and shoe to the pedal. This was a tremendous advantage over the traditional pedals, on which you could only push down. Toe clips allowed power to be transferred in every part of the pedal stroke. A down side to this style was that it took quite a bit of effort to get out of them when preparing to stop.

The "clipless" pedal resolved this issue by attaching a cleat to the bottom of the shoe, which would then clip into the pedal. This became known as the clipless pedal, replacing toe clips as the best way to secure a rider's shoe to the pedal. They became known as clipless pedals, even though this new technology involved clipping into the pedal. Safety was also enhanced, because a simple twist of the foot could release the shoe from the pedal.

Clipless pedals take a little getting used to and you should practice clipping and unclipping many times while holding on to a couch or some other stable base before trying them on the road. Then, when heading out on the road, make a conscious effort to remind yourself to unclip at least 10 yards before you need to stop. Just unclip whichever foot you plan to put down, but do it early so when it's time to actually stop, it's just a matter of placing your foot on the ground. I cover this in some detail because most new riders, including myself, have tipped over when coming to a stop as a result of not unclipping. After several years, I now find unclipping to be second nature.

Back to the pedal stroke. Now that you can clip and unclip safely, there are some simple drills you can do while riding to help develop a more powerful pedal stroke by using more muscles to create power. After a good warm-up, when the pedal starts coming forward, concentrate on pushing your foot forward in your shoe across the top of the pedal stroke. By doing this, you will engage parts of your quadricep muscle group that you otherwise won't use. Do this for 30 seconds and then pedal easily. After a little while, when the pedal starts moving backward, concentrate on pushing your heel to the back of your shoe through the bottom of the pedal stroke. By doing this, you will engage your hamstrings in a new way. Do this for 30 seconds and then pedal easily. Do two or three sets of these drills and then pedal easily for a while. Then, combine the two drills for two or three sets, each set lasting 30 seconds or so. Do these drills during one ride a week and you will significantly increase your power and efficiency.

Knee position is one of the most important areas we will discuss. Pro cyclists nearly brush the inside of their knees on the top tube of their bikes. Bob Forster has told me that although this may help with a slight power increase for professional riders, non-professionals should not use this technique, as it tends to cause knee problems. Accordingly, for proper form for non-pros, knees should be in the same plane as hips and ankles, allowing for the safest and most efficient transfer of power.

For more specific tuning of your pedal stroke, see a physical therapist who specializes in cycling, or go to a cycling coach. Spinscan, which is the software used by Computrainer, is a fantastic tool to help identify and correct some issues in a pedal stroke. When I got serious about triathlon training, I went to a cycling specialist named Andrew Gonzales at Kilowatt Cycling. Andrew used the Spinscan feedback to fine-tune my pedal stroke. Go to my website to connect with Andrew.

6. Mechanics of Freestyle Swimming

SWIMMING IS ONE OF THE MOST TECHNIQUE-DEPENDENT OF ALL sports. This is because water creates more resistance against your body than air. It is estimated that a 10% increase in efficiency in a swim stroke will result in an 11% improvement in speed, while a 30% increase in power will result in only a 10% improvement in speed. This means there is a much greater reward for efficiency through proper swimming form when compared to an increase in power. Of course, ideally, the goal should be to increase both efficiency and power.

I see many new swimmers, and especially men, swim like a board being pulled horizontally along the surface of the water. You can see the backs of both shoulders at all times with their arms just barely lifted out of the water as they move them forward to start the next pull. These same swimmers also have feet which are very deep in the water, creating a tremendous amount of drag. Because they keep their heads up while they swim, their hips and legs are pushed down.

Conversely, good mechanics create a balanced stroke, which puts shoulder, hips, and feet at the surface along with a balanced rotation, creating the longest and strongest stroke possible. Good mechanics will also create the smallest hole possible in the water through which to pull your body.

Head position: Other than taking a breath, the back of your head is the only part of it which should be above the surface. As you rotate, proper head position will keep your neck straight, allowing your mouth to come to the surface to take a breath. Exhale when your face is in the water so you can spend as much time as possible inhaling when your mouth is in position to take a breath.

Torso: you want your torso to be taut, meaning it may rotate, as if on a rod passing through the top of your head and exiting through the bottom of your feet, and your torso should not have a lot of "wiggle." When recently getting some coaching from Gerry Rodrigues, owner of Tower 26 swim coaching, he described some of my body motion as being similar to a semi truck with two trailers under heavy braking. When a tractor pulling a couple of trailers applies heavy brakes, the trailers do not stop in a perfectly straight line behind the tractor. In fact, they tend to go slightly different directions. This is what I looked like in the water, as a result of overextending my reach. I was bending from side to side at my waist, and was very inefficient. He explained that I should keep my torso long and taut, with very little wiggle in my mid-section. I clarified by asking if he wanted me to look more like a bullet train, with everything tracking straight, instead of looking like a semi tractor trailer rig under heavy braking. He paused for a moment, giving it careful thought, and then agreed.

Shoulders should rotate about 30 degrees from the surface of the water, and the hips should rotate a little less. During this rotation, when the hand is completely extended, it should be directly in front of your shoulder on that side. When reaching forward, make sure to lengthen your reach by allowing your shoulder to extend forward. With the arm fully extended you are now ready to "catch" the water and start your pull. As the hand enters the water, you want the thumb and index finger to enter first. You also want the hand relaxed, and a little separation between the fingers. As you begin to pull, hand and forearm should be in a straight line, your fingers should be pointed down, while keeping your elbow high. This creates the largest surface area possible to pull or push against the water. Pull your hand and forearm straight back, without crossing the centerline of your body. If your hand crosses your body's centerline, you are pulling and pushing laterally, which is very inefficient. You want to pull straight back, almost like when you climb a ladder, so your hand ends up next to your hip at the finish of the stroke. Swim coaches talk about high elbows during the pull phase, which means keeping them relatively close to the surface of the water. This means that as you pull, you don't want to keep your arm straight and rotate only at the shoulder like a windmill. A proper swim stroke involves a bend at the elbow, which allows the hand to remain close to the body, allowing for the most efficient motion.

Hips: as the shoulders rotate, so should the hips. As you finish a stroke and your hand approaches the hip on that side, the hip should be rotating toward the surface.

Legs and feet: the type of swimming you do will determine how much kick you use. If your plan is to race in a pool over shorter distances, then more kicking will probably be better. However, if you plan to do more endurance swimming or prepare for a triathlon, then it will probably be best to kick a little less, and save energy for the bike and run. A proper kick happens just below the surface, with just a slight bend at the knee. Your heel can break the surface of the water, but if your entire foot comes out and then re-enters the water, creating a splash, you need to concentrate on a little more hip angle or a little less knee deflection to keep your feet in the water. Your feet can't push you forward if they are not in the water.

One way to think of efficient swimming is to think of creating a small hole in the water with your hands, head, and shoulders and then pulling the rest of your body through that hole. The smaller you can make the hole, the more hydrodynamic you will be, which will result in greater speed because of reduced resistance.

7. Getting a Coach

COACHING, LIKE UNDERGOING TESTING TO DETERMINE YOUR EXact heart rate zones, involves some expense. However, the benefit from good coaching will both decrease the chance of injury and enhance performance with reduced exertion as a result of improved mechanics. If you aren't moving properly, your mechanical efficiency will be poor, which will prevent you from reaching your genetic potential. While the guidance I provide in this book is good, it may be difficult to reach your absolute maximum efficiency and potential without an expert watching you and correcting your specific issues.

Most of us have mechanics that are not perfect, so paying a coach who can help improve your mechanics can be a relatively small investment which can result in huge dividends. I spent one month swimming with Gerry Rodrigues and was 10 seconds faster over 200 meters: money well-spent. Good coaches can see mechanical issues you can neither see nor feel. A good coach will help your form, which will increase your speed and power, while also reducing the risk of injury.

It is also never too late to get a coach. Most if not all world champion athletes have coaches, because a coach can see flaws they can't. Also, this is not to say you will always need a coach. However, when getting started, it's a good idea to get a coach to make sure you are not building bad habits.

Finding a good coach may require a little research. Most areas of the country have master's swim teams, or cycling and running clubs that anyone can join for a small fee. Join one and find out who the best coaches are in the area by talking to members who have been in the sport for a while. Talk to a number of people to make sure you get a coach who will work best for your needs, schedule, and pocketbook.

You can also try what I call "spot coaching." This is when you hire a coach for a short period of time, for say one hour, and the coach will work with only you during that time. You will get feedback on what you need to work on for a few months on your own. Then, if you have improved in that area and want to improve more, have your coach take another look at you and give you new things to work on. You should work on improving only one or two things at a time, since most of us can't really concentrate on more than that at any one time.

I also want to offer a word of caution about coaches who were highly gifted athletes. In many cases, highly successful athletes are blessed with perfect genetics and they may have not utilized great training methodology to achieve their success. The point is, some of these great athletes, who do not know the methodology, pursue coaching careers following their competitive careers because they don't know anything else. Many people will use these coaches based on the coach's success as an athlete, without realizing they have limited knowledge of the best training principles.

When picking a coach, if you do your homework, you will be able to find one of the many great coaches who were also great athletes. However, there are a lot of great coaches who were never professional athletes, but they are still great coaches because they understand the methodology and have powerful observation and communication skills.

The art of coaching is seeing a flaw in form and then communicating how to correct the flaw to the athlete. Not everyone who calls themselves a coach can do both of theses things well. So, if you have a coach who doesn't see issues or communicate well, you probably need to keep looking. However, when you find a good coach, you will make corrections quickly, resulting in speed and strength increases.

8. MOTIVATION

STARTING ANY PROGRAM IS ALWAYS THE HARDEST PART. ONCE you have made the commitment to begin and then found which parts of this book will help you reach your goals, the greatest challenge will be making the time to do it. This means some of your previous activities may no longer be possible or may need to be modified to make time for this new focus. However, if you realistically assess what you do every day, you will likely find things you have done out of habit, which have collected over time and then trapped you in an unintended waste of time.

You may have noticed that I talk about balance a lot. That's because it is so important to leading a happy life. And like anything, to master it, you must understand it. Physical balance is accomplished by various large and small muscles working together to achieve a particular body position. In many cases, you may not even realize exactly which muscles are allowing you to achieve balance, because they are firing without conscious effort. If muscles fire with too much or too little intensity, or out of the necessary sequence, you can become out of balance and fall.

Similarly, in life, we achieve balance by the large and small parts of our lives working together, and if everything is weighted properly, peace and prosperity follow. Unlike some muscles, which may be small and deep inside our bodies and therefore unseen, everything in our day to day lives can be seen -- we simply need to look. The goal is to get rid of unnecessary parts of our day, as these things drain us of time and energy. By identifying the unnecessary parts of our day or week and replacing them with healthy eating and exercise, we can restore balance and lead a happier life.

Growing up with aspirations to be a professional football player, I watched a lot of football games, largely to learn how to play the game. This became a habit. By the time I graduated college and had my first real job, I had an epiphany one weekend as I was trying to squeeze into my weekend schedule things which were really important to me. The struggle came from the small amount of time left in the weekend after I watched two college football games on Saturday and two professional football games on Sunday. Those four games took up 12 hours of my weekend. I remember thinking that day that I was spending a huge amount of time watching football, and I didn't even have a favorite team. I then asked myself why I watched so much football.

This was an important question because it made me assess what I got out of watching the games. The answer was -- not much. I then realized I had fallen into this habit of watching large amounts of football and in doing so, I was wasting a great deal of time. It was a habit, which had grown over the years, and there really wasn't any reason for it. That day, I stopped watching football out of habit and then started watching only games in which I had a real interest. This change gave me back sometimes more than 10 hours a weekend.

Motivation begins with assessing and reassessing what you do in your day, and why. If you do an effective and honest assessment, you will likely find large windows of time available for healthy and productive activities. Then, when you find these windows, you must choose to make yourself and your health a priority.

Another important part of motivation is the ability to see how far you have come. Before you start this program, take a photo and put it somewhere you can see it regularly. Let the truth of the photograph of your old self serve as a continuing reminder of the changes you want to make. Also, get a complete physical, and with your doctor's approval, begin a program which includes proper nutrition, stretching, strength training, and cardiovascular exercise. Get another complete physical six or twelve months following the first one. Having these markers will serve as great motivation and help keep you on track and stay on whatever program you are following.

We are social animals, so join a gym. There are two main reasons for joining a gym. The first is: as social animals it is likely we will meet others in the gym who will serve as a support system. Simple camaraderie can easily be found in gyms, and other gym members will likely encourage you and could even go a step farther and become workout partners. The second reason to join a gym: just being around other people, whether interacting with them or not, we will usually try a little harder when someone else may be watching.

Back to the photo: when I was in the garage years ago and started strength training, I began seeing veins in my biceps for the first time. This provided great motivation for me. Seeing results is perhaps the strongest motivator. Once you earn the level of fitness and health you desire, through the use of a smart, sustainable program, motivation should never be an issue. As I always say, it is easier to stay in shape than it is to get into shape.

9. Injury Prevention

THE KEY TO INJURY PREVENTION IS EARLY DETECTION. TO DO THIS most effectively, you must listen to your body. That means if you feel soreness or tightness for two workouts in a row, treat it like an injury. Prior to reaching age 30 I was able to engage in almost any athletic activity, at maximum intensity, and as a result of my body's ability to quickly repair damage done during these exertions, I rarely sustained any serious injuries. In my early to mid-30s, that changed. As we get older, our body's ability to repair itself slows, which means more recovery time is needed between workouts.

Self-massage is the best way to detect issues early. In recent years I have been able to detect tightness in muscles, which I did not feel while stretching. Through what I call "scanning self-massage" I have found areas of tightness before I felt any other symptoms. I have then followed with focused cross-fiber massage on that specific area, followed by icing for 10 minutes. This practice has resolved most of my issues in only two to three days.

This strategy is essential for anyone who exercises regularly, because no matter how much you stretch muscles, they can still get tight. Scanning your muscles, by using your fingers to gently probe into the muscle, you can find areas which are tight. In more recent years, I have found many muscles which were just a little tighter than they should have been, and because I then did some deep cross-tissue massage on that area, the muscle loosened back up and I never became injured. If I had not developed this good habit of scanning my muscles regularly, I never would have found and treated these areas.

So, detecting tightness in a muscle or a part of a muscle is the best way to identify potential injuries. If you find areas that are tight, try some self-treatment as described above, and if that doesn't resolve the issue, see a physical therapist or your doctor.

DEEP TISSUE MASSAGE

Deep tissue massage, also known as cross-fiber massage, is a technique commonly used by physical therapists to loosen tight muscles, break up scar tissue, and increase blood flow in an injured part of the body. This can be painful, since tight muscles tend to be sore to the touch. The reality is, if a muscle is tight, pressure must be applied to loosen it up and help it heal. This is the most painful part of physical therapy, but is also perhaps the most important.

To find the precise spot of the injury, a physical therapist will dig around by applying pressure in different parts of a muscle or muscle group until they find the most painful spot. They will then continue to press and manipulate the area until it loosens up. This can be extremely painful, but the more pain you can stand, the deeper the massage can go. The deeper the massage can go, the faster the issue will heal. The extent of the injury, and the amount of pain you can tolerate, determine how many treatments you will need.

In addition to deep tissue massage, physical therapists will often use ultrasound on the area first. This puts heat deep into the tissue, allowing for a more pliable muscle, which allows the therapist to dig deeper. Following deep tissue massage, therapists will often use electro stimulation while icing. Electro stimulation involves small amounts of electricity passing through muscles, causing them to contract. Doing this with ice helps remove any waste products produced during deep tissue massage, and also helps increase blood flow in the area, which speeds up the healing process. Icing while receiving electro stimulation helps reduce any inflammation caused by the treatment.

Muscle Damage Causes and the Recovery Process

During higher exertions, or when doing new exercises, muscle fibers become damaged through micro-tears. These tiny tears are normal and are actually beneficial. The amount of damage is determined by the level of exertion, and how soon you begin the recovery process following the exertion. These micro-tears are also important because they trigger the body's adaptation response by increasing muscle fiber. The adaptation process is maximized only when proper nutrition and recovery time follow an exertion. When you don't allow the body time to adapt, by continuing with high exertions day after day, muscles can become very tight and inflamed, resulting in injury.

Understanding and following periodization allows the proper amount of damage to occur in muscles, allowing the body to adapt and get stronger instead of injured. The soreness and stiffness in the hours or days following high exertions or new exercises are the result of pain receptors inside the muscles, which are firing because of the micro-tears. When damage occurs inside the body, a normal response is inflammation. Inflammation is fluid sent to protect a damaged area. This inflammation, or swelling, inside the muscle can contribute to a muscle feeling stiff or tight, because of the additional fluid. The inflammation is directly related to the number of micro-tears.

You might think that once the exertion is completed, damage would stop occurring to the muscles. This is wrong, unless you begin recovering the right way. Following higher exertions, the body uses protein to repair the micro-tears and increase muscle fibers. If you don't consume protein, which puts it into your blood stream to be used by the muscles, your body will cannibalize itself by taking protein from another source in your body: existing muscles. This, of course, causes more damage.

However, with proper post-workout or race nutrition, you can minimize muscle damage and recovery time and actually increase muscle mass and strength. Following higher exertions, you have about 30 minutes to give your body what it needs in order to maximize your benefits. This is discussed more in the Post-Workout or Race Nutrition chapter.

WHEN TO SEE A DOCTOR AND/OR PHYSICAL THERAPIST

As mentioned earlier, the rule is: if an area is tight or sore for two workouts in a row, treat it like an injury. You can do deep tissue massage and ice at home and resolve most issues, if they are caught early enough. But if self-treatment does not resolve the issue, then you need to see a physician, preferably a sports medicine specialist. I prefer sports medicine specialists because they tend to be both more knowledgeable about injuries and how they occur, and they are also more empathetic to athletes who want to get healthy as soon as possible so they can get back to training.

I have a great orthopedic surgeon, Dr. Thomas Knapp. He has seen me through a number of injuries. When evaluating me, he checks for pain and mobility, he usually x-rays the area, and then if surgery is not needed, he prescribes physical therapy (PT). With a referral, most insurance companies will pay most of the cost of PT. With the exception of my shoulder issue which needed surgery, PT has resolved every injury I have ever had.

With many injuries, PT should be the first choice. But when PT does not resolve the issue and surgery becomes necessary, don't be afraid of it. I am thankful Dr. Knapp repaired my shoulder, and I am also grateful that during the follow-up PT, I learned proper stretching and strength training for my shoulder. Most of these techniques are included later in this book. Learning proper stretching and strength training is the reason my shoulders are stronger than they were before the surgery.

10. Perceived vs. Actual Exertion

WHEN IN HIGH SCHOOL AND COLLEGE, IN THE 1970S AND 1980S, the accepted coaching method involved having athletes run at a certain percentage of full speed. Running as fast as you could was considered full speed and 100% of your ability. So, if the coach called for 100% effort, you ran whatever distance was called for as fast as you could. But, since you can't sustain 100% effort for very long, coaches would have you run a little slower than full speed so you could run farther. For example, in order to maintain better form, the coach would have us run five 400-meter dashes at 80% effort, with a short rest in between each. This did make us stronger and faster. However, this was based on the perception that we were running at 80% of our full capacity. Were we really? Probably not.

Using perceived exertion in the 1970s and 1980s was fine, because that was all we had. The fact that so many coaches still use this method surprises me, especially regarding endurance sports. Many coaches and programs still have a scale with five or six points. Each point on the scale represents a level of exertion to be used during a given interval. While this is better than completely winging it, using perceived exertion is not the best way to train when running or riding.

The best way to train for endurance sports is with science and a heart rate monitor (HRM), to determine actual exertion. To know your actual exertion rate, which is identified by your pulse ranges, you must get either a BLT or VO2 test. These tests allow you to exercise in the proper pulse ranges called for in periodization, and maximize your training benefit.

Perceived vs. Actual Exertion

These tests identify precisely when you produce more lactic acid than your body can process, or anaerobic threshold (AT). Knowing your AT, and exercising at or near it at the right time, improves your body's ability to process lactic acid, thus allowing you to run or ride faster for longer, and without the risk of "bonking." Bonking refers to a condition that occurs to some endurance athletes in the latter stages of races, when the ability to continue becomes severely compromised. This is usually the result of overexertion, poor nutrition, poor hydration or a combination of all three.

With a HRM you can also follow a race pulse protocol and never again worry about bonking as a result of overexertion. You can further ensure you never bonk again by following the nutrition and hydration guidance in this book.

11. BLT vs VO2 Max

BLT

THE BLT MEASURES THE AMOUNT OF LACTIC ACID, KNOWN AS lactate, produced by your muscles during exercise. The test is conducted either on a treadmill or bike and the speed or resistance is increased every four minutes. Just before the speed is increased a pinprick blood sample is taken from one of your fingers and the amount of lactic acid in your blood is measured. This test provides a very precise measurement of lactic acid in the blood in the various pulse ranges.

VO2 Max Testing

VO2 Max testing measures the maximum volume of oxygen you uptake, and provides additional information over the BLT; however, this test measures the composition of the air you exhale, thus eliminating the need to take blood samples. VO2 tests also measure which fuel source, or combination of fuel sources you use, and also measures the calories being burned in each pulse zone. The protocol is similar to the BLT, but you wear a mask, which captures the air you exhale. Like the BLT, the speed or resistance is increased every few minutes and your heart rate is recorded, to establish your various pulse thresholds.

Although I provide anecdotal guides to identify your base pulse range and your AT, these guidelines could be off enough to make a dramatic difference in the gain you would make if using the actual numbers. For instance, if you are running as much as 10 beats per minute (bpm) faster than your actual base pulse range, you could be burning 50% less fat compared to the amount you would burn if you were actually in your base pulse range.

Such testing is a bargain compared to what they cost 10 to 20 years ago. 20 years ago, only elite athletes used them, as they cost $1500 to $2000. Today, these tests should cost only $150 to $200. You should also retest periodically to determine how much you have improved and, because of your improved cardiovascular fitness, what your new pulse zones are. Most testing facilities will reduce their rates if you pay for several tests. Go to my website to find a facility.

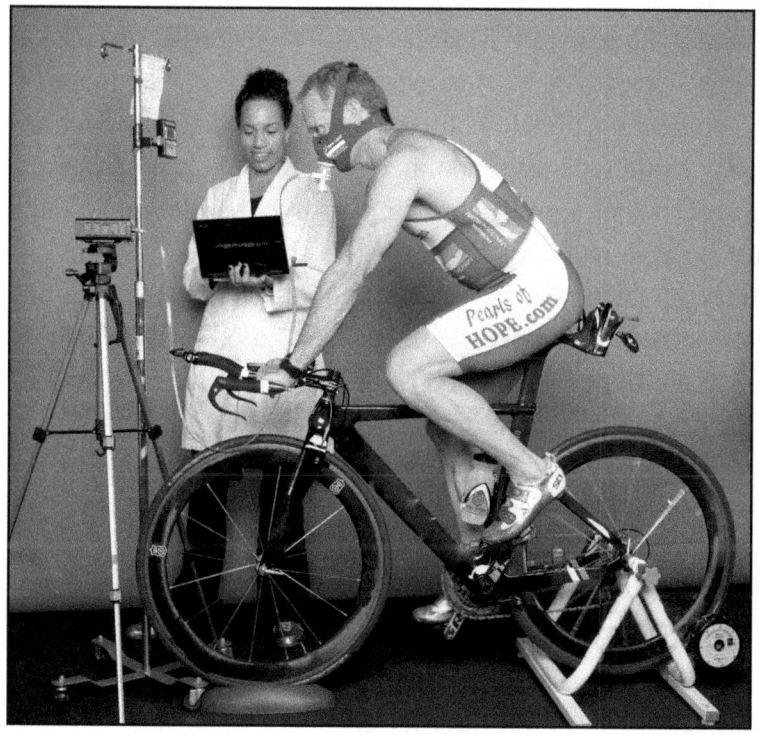

Photo by: Felicity Murphy

Exercise Physiologist Aishea Maas giving me a New Leaf VO2 test on my bike at Phase IV.

The use of these tests are also why I recommend you don't over-data yourself with most of the information you can get from many HRMs or bike computers during each training session. Downloading every workout and combing through the data can be counterproductive. If you are trying to identify your baseline, that's one thing, but if you are looking for improvement in each mile of each workout, you will likely become frustrated because you will probably not be able to see it, for a variety of reasons. Meaningful improvements occur over months and years, not days.

Unless you are an elite athlete, looking at all of the numbers most HRMs and bike computers provide for each mile of each workout, will probably frustrate you. For example, if you look at the time it took you to ride a particular mile on Wednesday, and then compare the time it took you to ride the same mile the previous Monday, you may be disappointed if Wednesday's time was slower. However, if you consider the three-to-five-mile-an-hour headwind you may have had to ride into Wednesday, which was not present Monday, it would make sense. Such slightly different conditions can be very difficult to perceive, unless you are actually watching the trees. Accordingly, if you don't notice the difference in conditions, you will likely conclude the reason you were slower Wednesday compared to Monday was because you did not have as much power. This could lead to needless confusion and frustration. Even if you notice the wind, quantifying its speed and how it might affect you will be almost impossible. So the keys are: know what pulse range you should be in, and be in it, while also making sure your cadence is in the 90 range, regardless of how fast you are going.

So, stay focused on the best guides of pulse and cadence and don't overdata yourself on a daily basis. It takes about three months to reprogram your physiology, so it won't be possible to see meaningful changes on a daily basis. Get tested so you have your numbers, and don't look at time or pace while exercising -- look just at your pulse. Stay in whatever pulse zone is called for in that workout. Then, measure your fitness every six months by getting another VO2 test or BLT, to find out what your actual improvement is. This testing will not only quantify your actual improvement, it will identify your new pulse zones based on that improvement.

I recommend a similar strategy regarding body weight, nutrition, and hydration. Instead of trying to measure every gram of carbohydrate, protein, and fat you eat, you should follow the directions in the Eating Program. First, get an idea of what you are eating and what is in it, by mapping what you eat every day for a week, then weigh yourself every day at the same time to monitor any changes in your weight. In doing so, you will be able to identify eating habits that are problematic, and those you should keep. I have a similarly simple method to monitor hydration.

In summary, keep it simple and don't overdata yourself on a daily basis. Trust and follow the program, and get a VO2 or BLT test periodically to determine the impact the program is having on your fitness, and get an annual physical to see the impact on your health.

12. Tailoring Your Program

TAILORING A PROGRAM TO YOUR SPECIFIC GOALS AND LIFESTYLE will require some education and commitment. Regardless of which cardiovascular exercise or combination of cardiovascular exercises you choose, the stretching and strength-training programs below will be essential to maximize fitness. In order to promote full-body fitness, all of the stretching and strength-training exercises will help you obtain better flexibility, mobility, and strength, while greatly reducing the risk of injury.

Stretching should take only about five minutes before and after each workout, and the complete strength-training program should take only about one and a half to two hours a week. If you strength train three days a week, that's 30 minutes each workout. If your goal is to put on a little more muscle, your strength-training program will need to be a little longer, since in this case I recommend three sets of each exercise instead of two. If you want to gain muscle even faster, stength train each body part twice a week instead of once, but don't work the same body part two days in a row.

Whichever cardiovascular exercise you choose, I recommend at least 30 minutes three times a week. If you are interested in burning more fat, 60 minutes three times a week at a low heart rate is much better. As a rough guide, if you want to increase your workout time, you can safely add 10 to 15% a week, and then reduce your volume by 40 to 50% each fourth week, which will be your recovery week.

13. STRETCHING

BOB FORSTER SAYS, "IF YOU DON'T HAVE TIME TO STRETCH BEfore and after each workout, you don't have time to workout." It is really important to adopt this philosophy. Even though we didn't have periodization as a workout guide when I ran track and played football, we still stretched. I credit a good stretching program with allowing me to train and race into my 30s. I improved my stretching program as I learned the best ways to safely stretch during my many years as a physical therapy patient.

Stretching increases mobility and blood flow, both of which are needed prior to exercise in order to help prevent injury and maximize performance. If you are particularly tight in one or more areas of your body, you should think about stretching several times a day, even if you don't plan to work out.

Improving mobility through stretching is a gradual process. Each time you stretch, if you do so properly, you will improve by becoming a little more flexible. Over the course of months, the improvement might be only another few degrees of range of motion. However, improvement -- no matter how slight -- is still improvement, and that improvement will continue until you reach your maximum functional flexibility, as long as you continue to stretch properly.

Stretching has been highly misunderstood for a long time. There has been a lot of debate about what type of stretching to do, for how long, and when. There are even a few voices that say stretching can hurt performance, but this is wrong if the stretching is done correctly. The stretching protocol in this book is the one I use and teach. Everyone I have coached with it has seen improvements in flexibility and performance.

So, although stretching is good, there are some things you should never do, like bounce when stretching. Bouncing while stretching dramatically increases the likelihood of injury while stretching. When you bounce while stretching, you create a reflexive contraction of the muscle you are trying to stretch. This means that while you are applying pressure to make the muscle longer, the muscle quickly contracts, making it shorter, which can result in an injury in the form of a strain or pull. You should also never have someone push on you when you stretch. This can easily result in overstretching and cause injury. Physical therapists or trainers who are experts will sometimes push on an athlete to maximize a given range of motion. However, these are experts working on highly trained athletes. For the rest of us, it will be far better to stretch regularly, using the system below, and be happy with the gradual increases in flexibility we will attain.

Proper stretching involves applying just enough pressure so you can feel a little tension in the muscle being stretched, but there should not be any pain. Hold the stretch for eight to ten seconds, gradually release, and do it one more time. Twice each side for eight to ten seconds per stretch is all you need. Many of the leg stretches in the program are performed lying on the ground, in order to protect the lower back and increase stability.

STRETCHES:

LEGS
GLUTEALS
PRETZEL

Lying on your back, cross your legs as you might when sitting in a chair, with the lower part of a leg across the knee of the other. Place your hands on the back of the leg which is straight up just below the knee. While keeping your hips on the floor, pull the knee toward your chest. You should feel the stretch in your bottom.

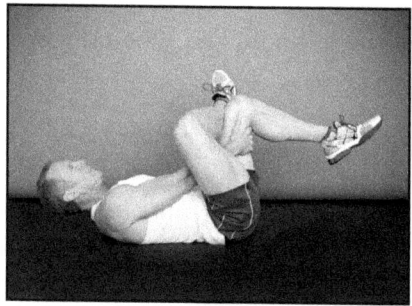
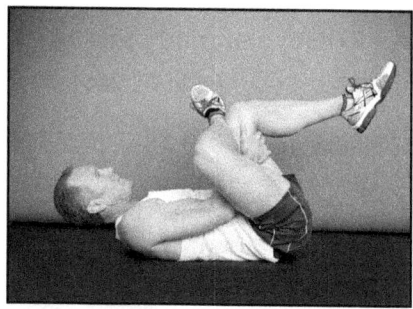

Photos by: Felicity Murphy

Start   Finish

FIGURE 4

Now we are going to increase hip mobility. While in the pretzel position, place one hand on top of your ankle and the other hand on the inside of the knee of that leg. The hand, which is holding your ankle, will be a pivot point for this stretch. Now, holding your ankle in place, with the hand on your knee, gently start pushing your knee away from you. You should feel a stretch deep inside the hip. If you feel any pain in your knee during this stretch, stop and consult a physician or physical therapist.

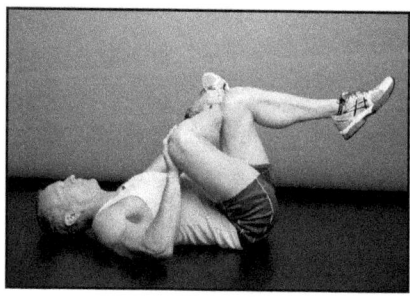
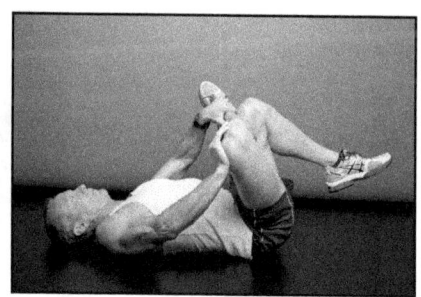

Start   Finish

THE FROG

Lying on your back, slide your feet toward your butt, and let your knees flare out. Place the palms of your hands on the inside of your knees and gently press down on your knees. You should feel a stretch on the inside of your thigh.

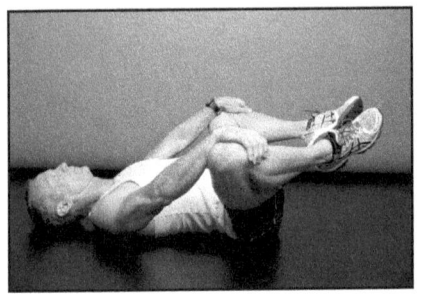 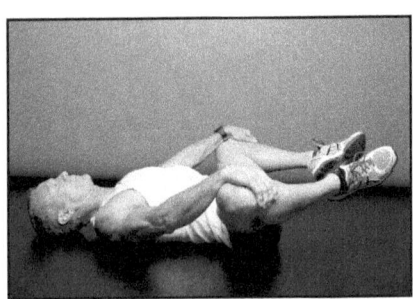

Start   Finish

HAMSTRINGS

Lying on your back, maintain a slight bend in your knee and pivoting at the hip joint, raise one leg as high as you can. With both hands, grasp as high on your leg as possible. If you can't reach your leg with your hands, you can use a strap or towel and put it over the bottom of your shoe and gently pull your foot toward your head. You should feel a stretch in the back of your upper leg.

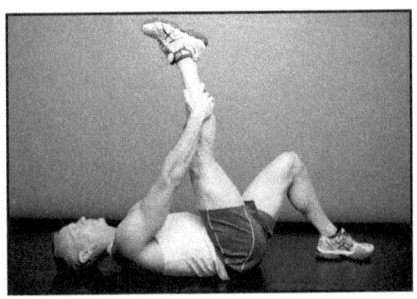 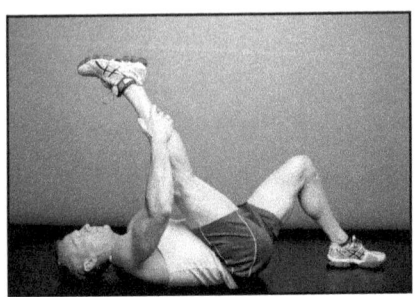

Start   Finish

QUADRICEPS

While lying on your side, bend the "top" leg at the knee and grasp your ankle with your hand. Keeping your thigh parallel with the floor, gently pull on your ankle. You should feel a stretch in the front of your upper leg.

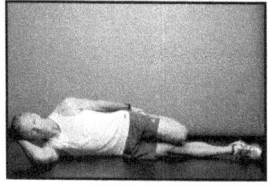 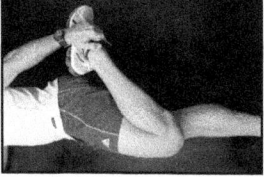 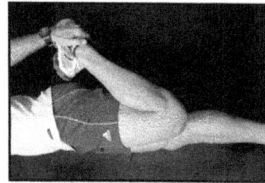

Front Start View   Start Top View   Finish Top View

HIP FLEXOR

In a kneeling position, with one knee up and one knee down and your torso proudly vertical, keep your shoulders in the same place and gently rotate your hips forward. You should feel the stretch in the front of the hip of the down leg.

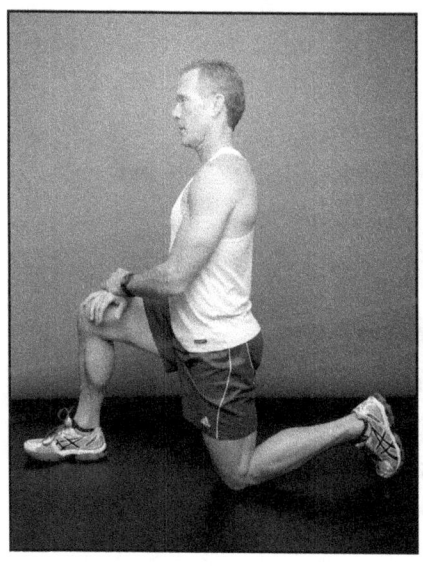 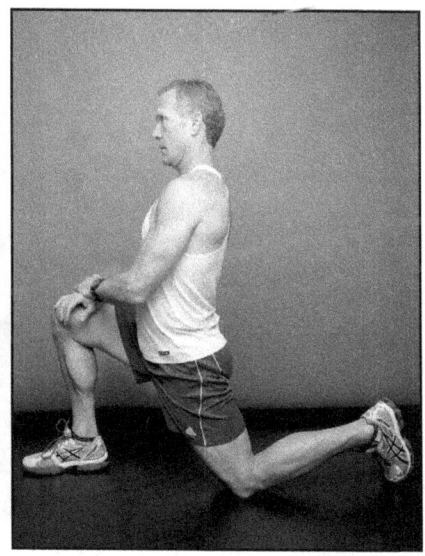

Start   Finish

CALVES

GASTROCNEMIUS

With your feet shoulder width apart, lean forward and place both hands on a wall, keeping your arms straight. While keeping your heels on the ground slowly lower yourself toward the wall by bending at the elbow. You should feel a stretch at the back of your leg, which runs from behind the knee into the upper calf.

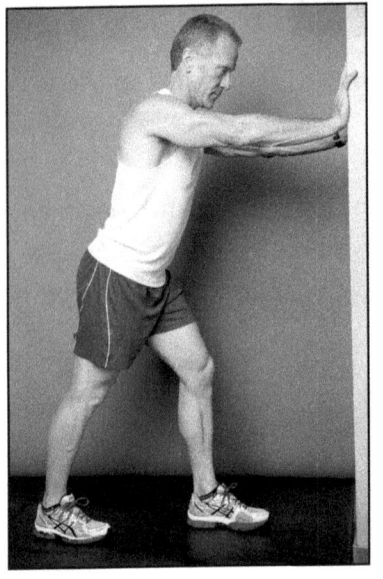
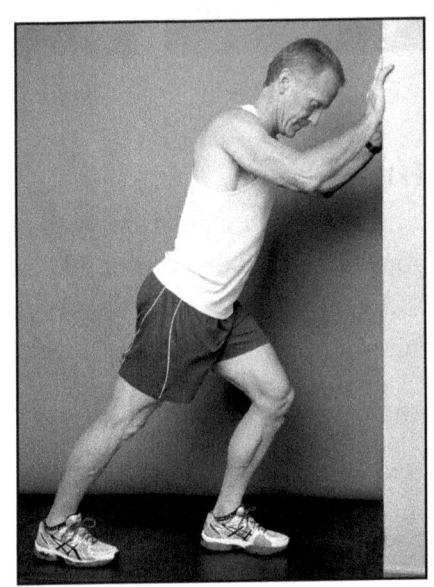

Start   Finish

SOLEUS

This is the second big muscle in the calf and is often overlooked. It fires when the knee is bent, which is why we must stretch and strengthen it with a bent knee. I like to combine this stretch with the gastrocnemius stretch. So, after doing that one, I straighten my arms, bend one knee and lower myself toward the wall. You should feel the stretch in the lower part of the calf in your back leg.

STRETCHING

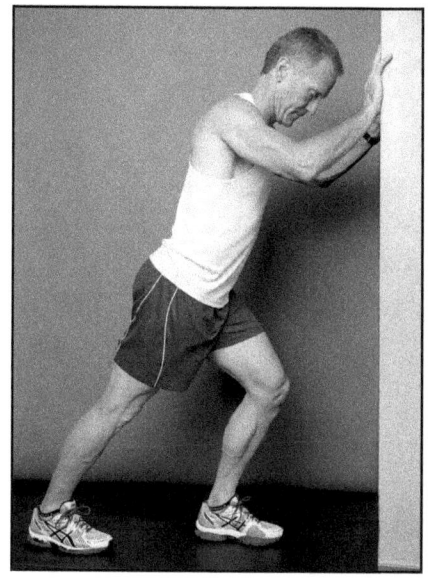
Start

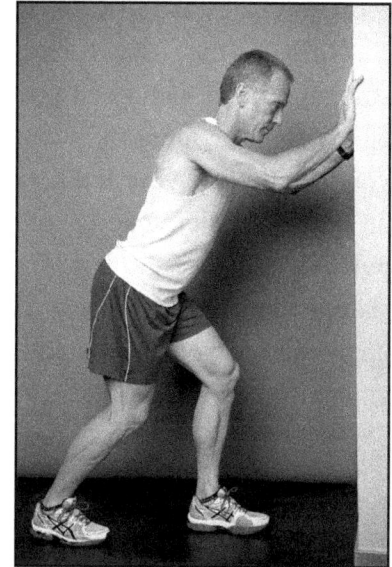
Finish

SHOULDERS/CHEST/BACK

REAR DELTOIDS

Extend one arm so it is in front of you and then rotate it so it is across your chest. Place the hand of your other arm on the back of the elbow, which is across your chest, and gently pull your elbow into your chest. Keep the elbow of the arm being stretched low, and you should feel the stretch at the back of your shoulder.

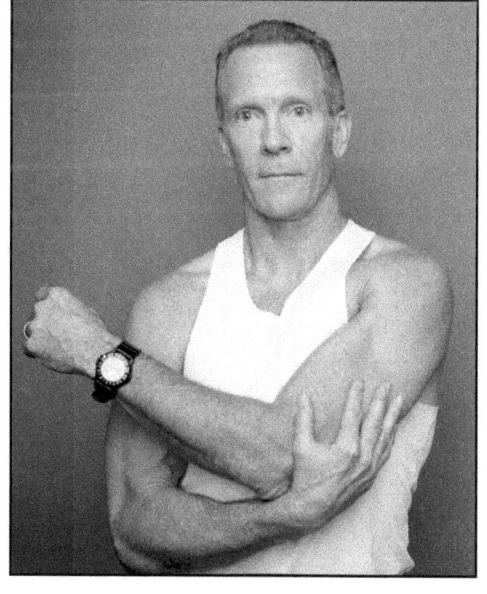

TRICEP/LATISSIMUS DORSI

Raise your right arm straight up and then bend your elbow so your forearm is over your head. Place your left hand on your bent elbow and gently pull the elbow to the left. You should feel the stretch on the upper side of your back and in your tricep.

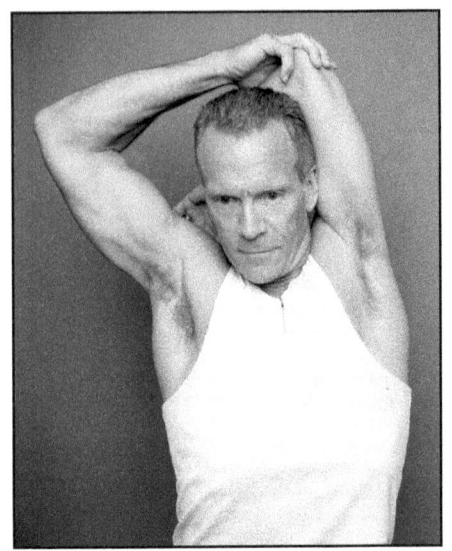

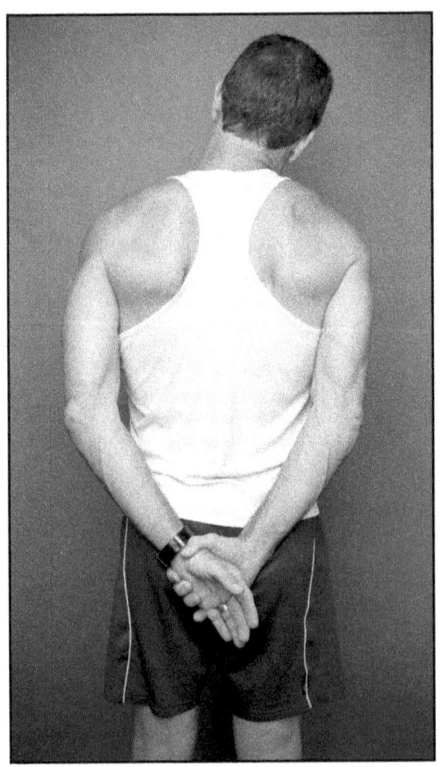

TRAPEZIUS

Put your right hand in the small of your back and grasp at the wrist with the left hand. Using your left hand, gently pull your right arm toward the ground. You should feel a stretch at the base of your neck. To increase the effect, tilt your head away from the side you are stretching.

CHEST

Using the corner of a wall or a doorway, place your hand about shoulder level. Place the foot nearest the wall slightly in front of you. Keep your head up and gently put some weight on your front foot. This will rotate your torso slightly and you should feel the stretch in your chest.

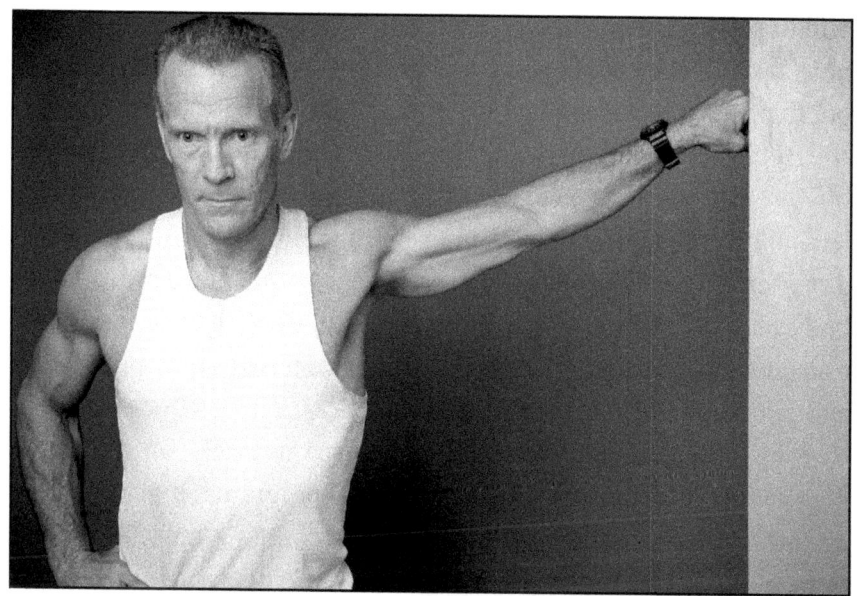

14. Strength Training

THIS PROGRAM WILL NOT MAKE YOU A "BODY BUILDER." BODY builders spend many hours each day lifting weights and usually must take all sorts of illegal and unhealthy drugs and supplements to build massive muscles that have little athletic function.

By contrast, although this program will improve strength and build some muscle, the strength you will gain will improve your athletic ability. Combine this strength-training program with some cardiovascular exercise and a proper eating program, and a reduction in body fat will result in a lean and sculpted body with improved function and better speed. You will also improve testosterone production and circulation throughout your body.

This strength-training program focuses not only on the larger muscles worked in most strength-training programs, it also focuses on the smaller stabilizer muscles. These stabilizing muscles are extremely important for proper function and also play a significant role in injury prevention. They are also small muscles that most strength training programs don't focus on, and which high-intensity exercise regimens, which use gross body weight for resistance, can't strengthen properly.

For example, we will work on the rotator cuff, a collection of tendons that connect the deltoid muscles to the upper arm bone (humerus). They are deep inside the shoulder and are critical to shoulder function. Shoulder function is important because it is critical to all arm movement. As a result of a general weakness in the rotator cuff, many athletes who throw things get injured. In many cases, these injuries could have been prevented with proper stretching and strength training of some very unglamorous but very important muscles.

You will probably be familiar with many of the exercises in this program; however, I suspect you will see a few new ones. Also, this program uses lighter weights than most programs. That's because many of the exercises focus on those small stabilizer muscles, which are so important to function. Also, the reality is that you don't need to lift super-heavy weights to become functionally strong.

We will use lighter weights so we can focus on proper form. It is better to do an exercise properly with a little less weight than it is to do an exercise incorrectly with a little more weight. So, look closely at the example photos and read the description of the exercise to be sure you are doing it correctly. Start with light weights for each exercise, and carefully assess the movement. If you feel any pain, stop and double check to make sure you are doing it correctly. If you are doing the exercise correctly and still experience pain, stop doing that exercise and check with your doctor to see if you have a pre-existing injury.

Let me also stress the importance of core work. I call it core work instead of an ab routine, because abs refer to just the abdominal muscles and obliques on the front of your body. Abs can be great show muscles, and are often worked vigorously and to the exclusion of the muscles in the lower back region.

By contrast, the term core refers to the development of the abdominal, obliques, and lower back muscles, resulting in proper balance. Your pelvis has four major muscle groups pulling on it: quadriceps, hamstrings, abdominals, and lower back. Having flexibility and strength in those four muscle groups literally provides balance. If you lack strength and flexibility in any of these areas, you will be out of balance. Such imbalance can lead to injury, most commonly in the lower back. A proper core-strength-training program coupled with a good stretching program can help prevent or correct many lower back issues.

Also, given the 39 years I have been strength training, I have done most exercises and made a lot of mistakes, many of which have led to injury. However, I have learned from those mistakes. The strength-training program in this book is designed to improve strength while preventing injury. The exercises in this book are guided by Bob Forster, who has decades of experience regarding what are the right and wrong exercises. Over the years, Bob has seen exercise trends that cause injuries. His experience is a heavy guide for the exercises I recommend.

As a result, you may notice a few classic weight-lifting exercises are not included in this program. I do not recommend doing squats, military press, "dips," or leg extensions, as these all have a strong correlation with causing injuries. Squats are known to contribute to knee and lower back issues, military press and dips have a high correlation with causing shoulder impingement, and leg extensions are known to cause irreparable damage to the back of the patella (knee cap).

Instead of squats, I recommend a seated leg press. It works the same muscles as squats but protects the lower back and knees, when done correctly. We won't do any shoulder exercises that press the weight overhead. Instead, we will do a number of shoulder exercises, raising the weight to shoulder height or just a little above.

The number of repetitions is determined by what phase you are in. For base phase, use lighter weights and do two sets of 20 repetitions. During the building phase, add a little weight and do two sets of 15 repetitions. For peak phase, increase the weight a little more and do two sets of 10 repetitions.

The number of sets I normally do and recommend in this program is two per exercise, working each body part once a week. However, if your goal is to put on a little more muscle in a given area, you can add a third set. If your goal is to put more muscle on faster, then you can strength train each body part twice a week, but

Strength Training

don't work the same body part two days in a row.

Choose weights that allow you to complete a set relatively easily. This means, if you are doing a set of 20 repetitions you should be able to do 23 or 25 if you needed to. If you use weights that allow you to just barely complete the set, you will likely start to "cheat." Cheating means you are using non-targeted muscles to complete the motion. This can lead to injury. Make sure the weights you use allow you to complete each set relatively easily without cheating. Think about which muscles you are using for each exercise to help you achieve perfect form. If you can't complete a set perfectly, especially in the base phase, lower the weight and get it right.

Get a log and track the weights you use. There are a lot of exercises in this program, and until you have done it for a while it may be difficult to remember from week to week what weights you used for each. Go to my website for a link to a strength training log you can access at the gym with your smartphone.

I do each body part once a week, in four sessions, which take 30 to 45 minutes per session. The most efficient combination and sequence I have found is: day 1: legs, day 2: chest and back, day 3: shoulders, and day: 4 arms and core.

For legs, you may want to start doing the floor routine without ankle weights, and add ankle weights, starting with one pound once you have the movement down. Then, after you have progressed and reached the point where you can do five pounds easily, you may want to switch to doing the exercises using ankle straps on a cable machine. Go to my website for more information on ankle weights and ankle straps for cable machine exercises.

The term super-setting refers to doing more than one exercise at a time. This is a very time efficient way to strength train. For example, I like to super-set arms. I will do a set of a bicep exercise and then a set of a tricep exercise. While doing the tricep exercise the biceps are resting and they are ready for the next set when I finish the tricep set. The only issue with super-setting is that in a crowded gym you will be using more than one piece of equipment at a time. If someone wants to use one of the pieces of equipment you are using, which is usually indicated by them standing near the equipment and facing the equipment, a little communication can go a long way. Ask them if they are waiting for the equipment. If they are, tell them you are doing only two sets and consider inviting them to "work-in" with you. This means they can work on that piece of equipment while you are working on the other.

Always stretch before and after a strength or cardiovascular workout.

STRENGTH-TRAINING EXERCISES

LEGS

LEG PRESS

Seated in the leg press machine with feet about shoulder width, lower the weight or your body until you have a 90-degree angle in your knee. Going deeper than 90 degrees is widely known to cause knee injuries. This is the primary reason I don't recommend squats for strength training, since it is easy to go deeper than 90. With the leg press it is much easier to control how deep you go, and this exercise also protects your lower back compared to squats. Once you have the 90-degree bend in your knee, press the sled back to the starting position. Also, depending on your flexibility and range of motion, 90 degrees may be too deep. If that is the case, bring the weight down as deeply as you can comfortably and then press it back to the starting position. During the leg press, your knees should never go forward of your toes. To accomplish this, keep your feet in a position well in front of you when starting the exercise.

STRENGTH TRAINING

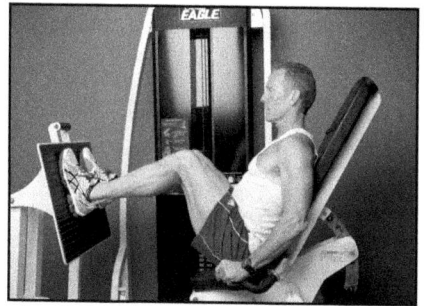 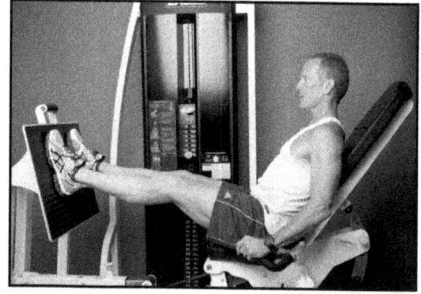

Photos by: Felicity Murphy

Start   Finish

STRAIGHT LEG CALF RAISES

While still seated in the leg press machine, adjust your feet so they are shoulder width apart, but your heels and arch are off the bottom of the platform. Press the sled up so your legs are straight. Then, using just your calf muscles, press the weight away from you with your feet so your toes are pointed away from you.

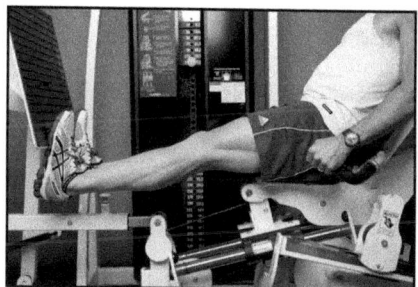 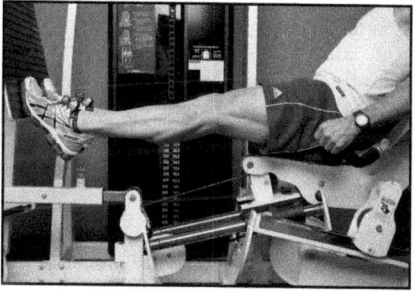

Start   Finish

HAMSTRING CURLS

We do these one leg at a time. When these are done with both legs, one leg is usually stronger and will do most of the work, leaving the weak leg vulnerable to injury. We eliminate this condition by using one leg at a time. Starting with the leg almost straight, bend at the knee and control the weight until your heel almost touches your butt.

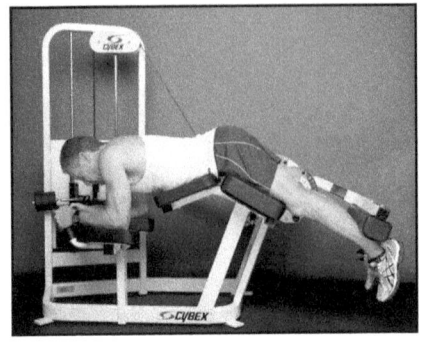 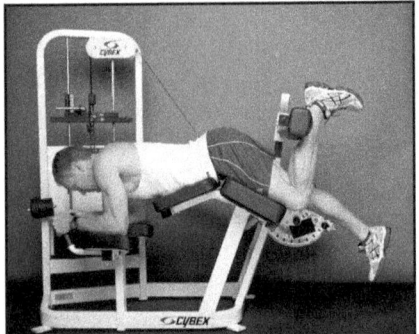

Start   Finish

SEATED CALF RAISES

Since the soleus, or lower calf muscle, fires best with a bent knee, we do bent-leg calf raises. If you don't have a seated calf raise machine, you can put weights on your knees to do the exercise. On a seated calf machine, place your knees under the pads and only the balls of your feet on the foot stand. Using only your calf muscles, raise the sled and clear the safety stop; then lower your heel as far as it will go and then lift your heel as high as it will go.

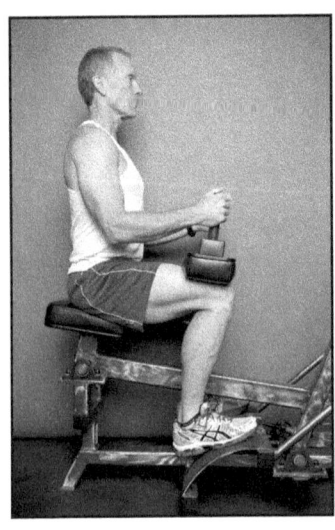 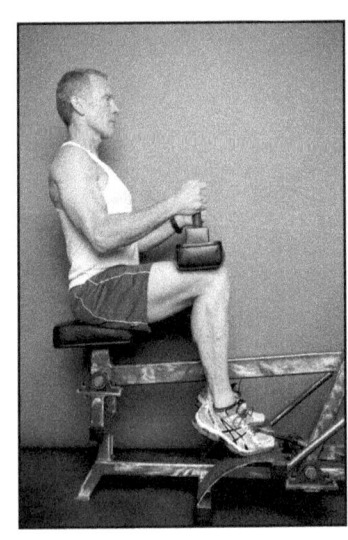

Start   Finish

Strength Training

Leg Cable Exercises

If you are just starting to exercise, you may want to do these exercises without any resistance. For beginners, the weight of your legs is enough to provide a good workout. When it becomes easy to do these exercises with just the weight of your legs, you may want to use adjustable ankle weights. Adjustable ankle weights are made of nylon, neoprene, and Velcro and have removable steel weights in them. They strap onto your ankles and you adjust the weight by removing or adding the steel weights. I recommend five-pound adjustable ankle weights and that you start with only one pound of weight. Add weight when the weight you have been using becomes easy. When the five-pound ankle weights become easy, you are ready to start using cable machines, or rubber fitness bands, which will require ankle straps.

I have done the research and found SPRI Products Inc. to make very high-quality adjustable ankle weights, ankle straps, and rubber fitness bands, among other fitness equipment. Visit my website for special offers and a link to SPRI.

Gluteus Maximus Extensions

While facing the machine and with the cable fastened to your ankle strap, keep a slight bend in your knee and move your foot away from the machine by rotating at the hip. You should not bend forward at the waist and you should not extend your leg too far back. I hold on to some part of the machine when I do these. This works

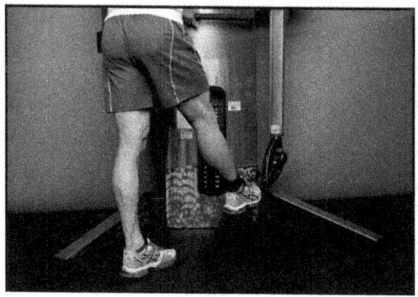
Start

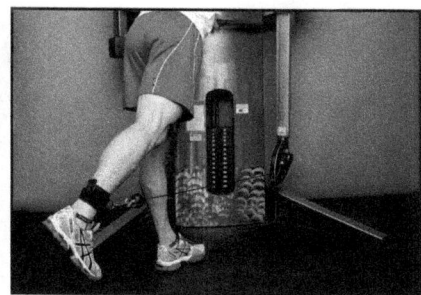
Finish

the largest of the three gluteal muscles, so I use the most weight on this exercise of all of the cable leg exercises.

ADDUCTOR - FRONT

With your body turned sideways to the machine and with the cable attached to the ankle closest to the machine, move your foot away from the machine with it passing in front of the foot on the ground. I hold on to some part of the machine when I do these.

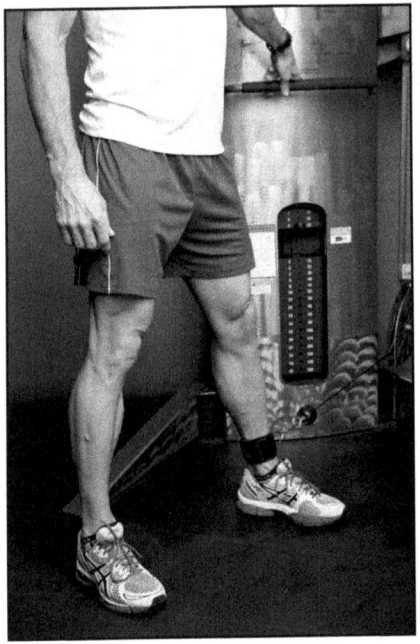 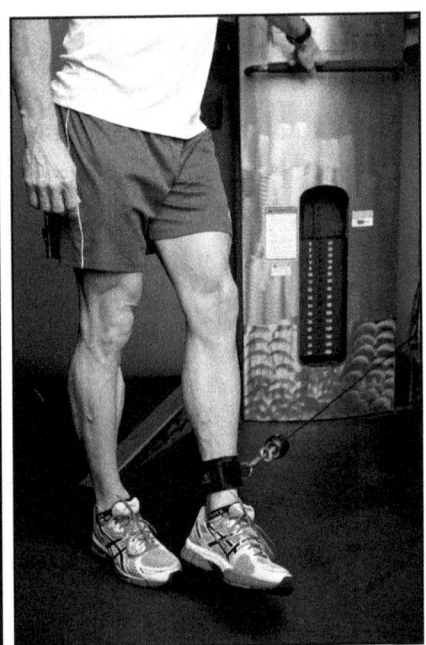

Start   Finish

HIP FLEXOR

With your body turned away from the machine, pull your knee up so it is as high as your waist. I usually do not hold on to anything when I do these, but it takes all my concentration to keep from falling over. If you need help balancing, find something to hang on to. I follow the Adductor - Front exercise with this because I use the same weight.

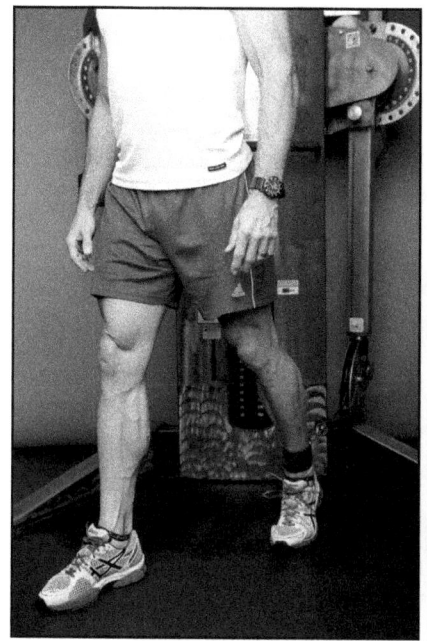
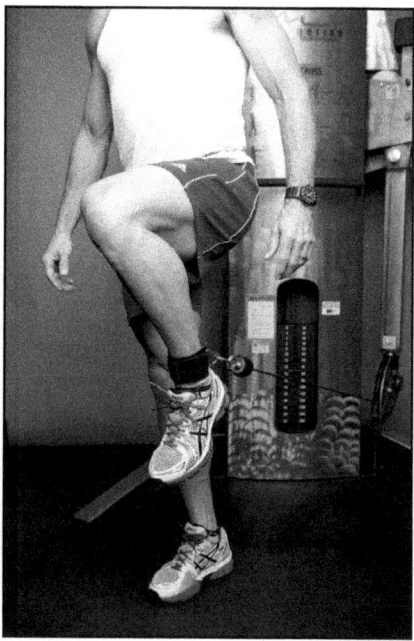

Start   Finish

ADDUCTOR - REAR

This is the same as the Adductor - Front exercise, but to the rear. With your body turned sideways to the machine, move your foot away from the machine with it passing behind the foot on the ground. I hold on to some part of the machine when I do these. Also, some people ask, why not do the front and rear exercises following each other? I like to work the Hip Flexor between the two to allow a little recovery between the Front and Rear Adductor exercises. Also, I use a little more weight when I do this exercise compared to the Front version.

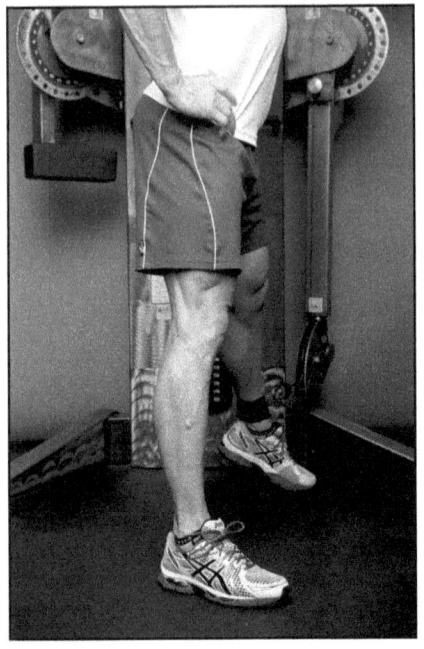 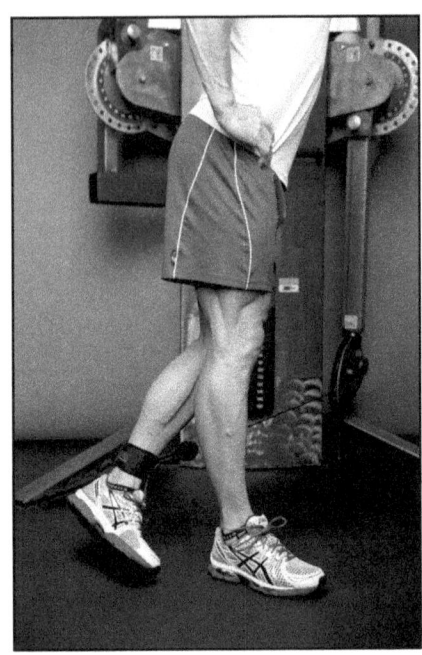

Start   Finish

Abductor

With your body turned sideways to the machine and the cable fastened to the strap on the outside ankle, move your foot away from the machine so you have a 20 to 30 degree angle between your legs. I hold on to some part of the machine when I do these. Also, I use the least amount of weight of all the cable leg exercises because the

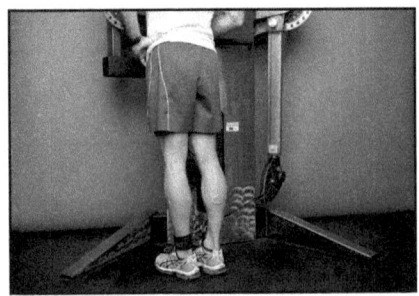 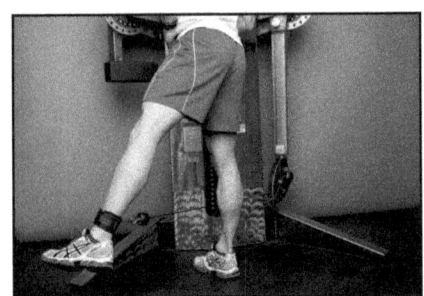

Start   Finish

primary muscles this exercise works are the gluteus minimus and gluteus medius, which are on the smaller side when compared to the gluteus maximus.

FLOOR LEG EXERCISES

For those just starting a strength-training program, it may be advisable to do the leg exercises above, but on the floor. To ensure you have the right range of motion, start these exercises without using ankle weights. Then, after a few weeks, add one pound every two weeks. Once you can do these exercises easily for two sets of 20 repetitions with five pounds on your ankles, you can add resistance by using an ankle strap with either a rubber fitness band fastened to a doorway or piece of furniture, or head to the gym and use a cable machine and very light weights.

GLUTEUS MAXIMUS EXTENSIONS

On your hands and knees, straighten one leg so it is in a straight line with your torso. Don't dip your torso by bending your arms, as this may cause you to over-extend the leg you are working. Keep your torso in the same position throughout the exercise and don't raise your leg too high. Raising your leg too high can put a lot of strain on your lower back.

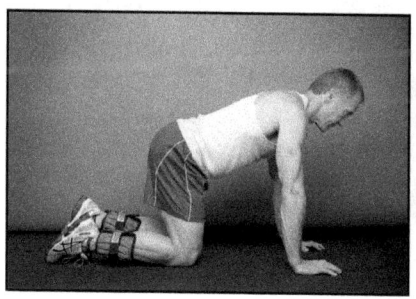
Start

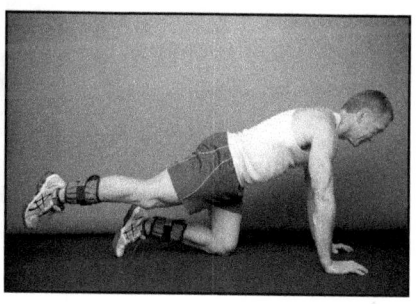
Finish

ADDUCTOR

While lying on your side, with your arm on the floor in front of you for stability, place the knee of your top leg on the floor in front of your body. Then move the leg on the floor up and behind your top leg.

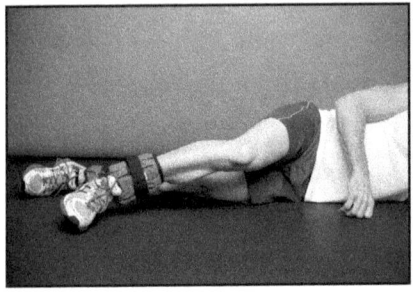
Start

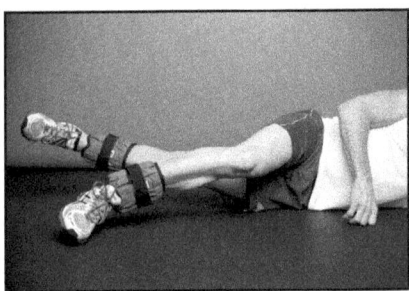
Finish

ABDUCTOR

Remaining on the ground on your side, your legs are straight and on top of each other. Raise the top leg so there are 20 to 30 degrees between them.

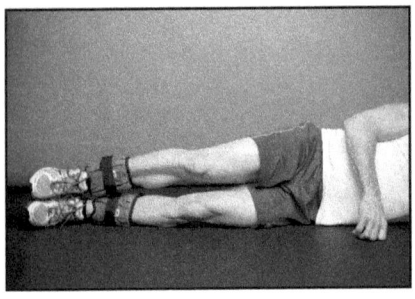
Start

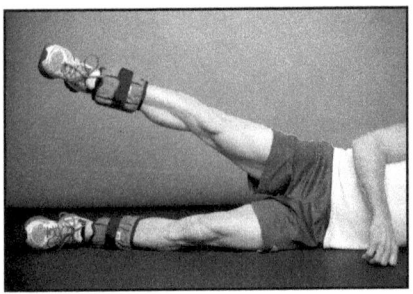
Finish

HIP FLEXOR

While standing and holding on to something for balance, raise one knee until it is even with your hip. This means your femur, or upper leg, will be parallel to the ground.

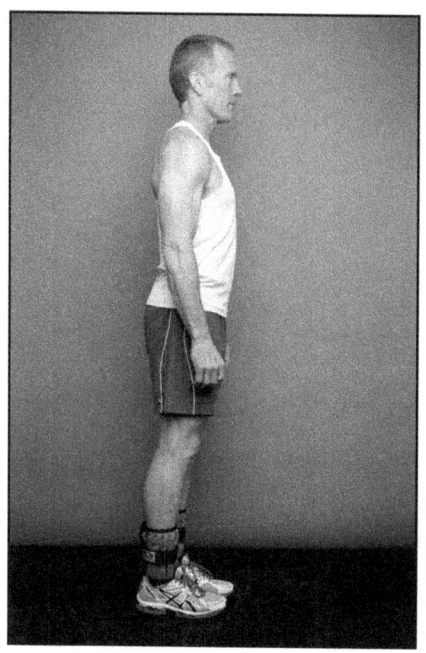 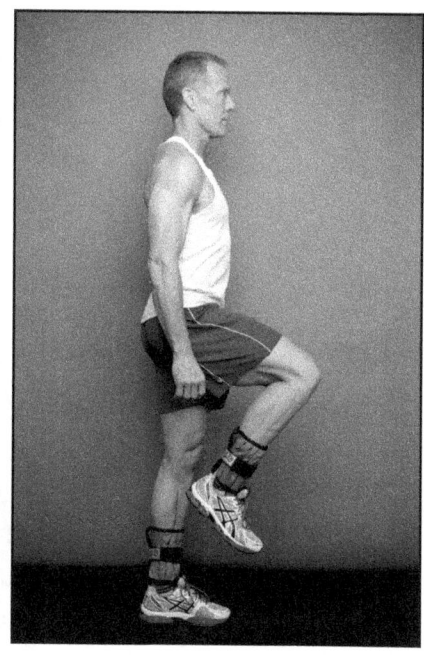

Start   Finish

SHOULDERS

Setting the shoulder: for shoulder or back exercises in which the starting position involves the weight hanging below your body, you will need to "set" your shoulder before starting the exercise. This means that while the weight hangs below you, your first movement is to pull your upper arm, the humerus, snugly into the shoulder socket with your rear deltoid and back muscles. It is a small movement, which protects the complex structure in your shoulders and also ensures proper function of an exercise.

REAR DELTOID EXTENSIONS

Either on a bench (to do one arm at a time) or standing and bent at the waist (to do both arms at the same time), a dumbbell is in your hand as it hangs below you. Set your shoulder, and then rotating at the shoulder and keeping your arm as straight as possible, move your hand back until your arm is parallel to the floor.

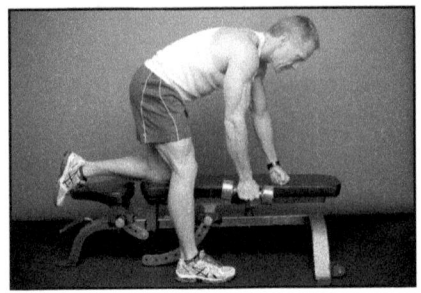 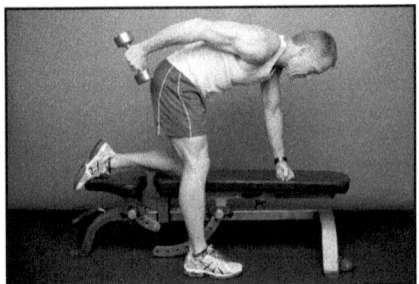

Start　　　　　　　　　　　　Finish

"Y" EXTENSIONS

While seated face down on an incline bench, with a dumbbell in each hand, set your shoulders and then rotate your arms forward at the shoulder to form the shape of a "Y." Your hands should come no higher than your shoulders.

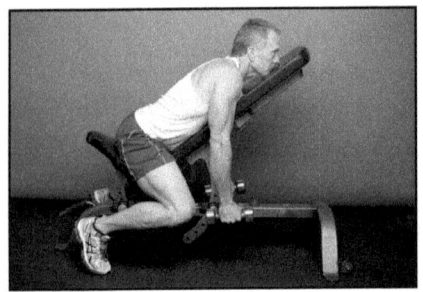 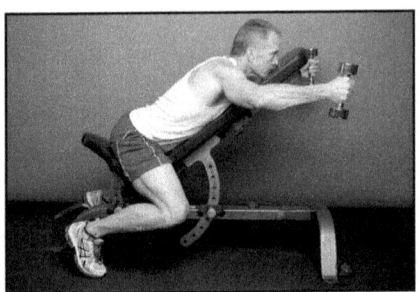

Start　　　　　　　　　　　　Finish

REAR DELTOID FLIES

Standing with a dumbbell in each hand, bend forward at the waist, keeping your back straight. Starting with the dumbbells hanging below you, set your shoulders and then rotate your arms out at the shoulder to bring your hands to shoulder height.

Strength Training

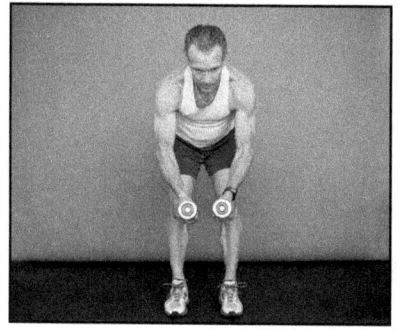 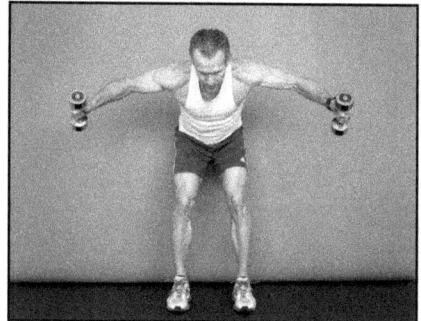

Start   Finish

Rotator Cuff Exercise Note

Note: Use very light weights for all of the rotator cuff exercises, as this area of the body is relatively delicate and complex. These exercises are designed to strengthen a number of tendons in the shoulder, which are not sufficiently strengthened by exercises focusing on the deltoid muscles. Although during peak phase training I can use as much as 40 pounds for some of these exercises, I have found that using weights like these can cause injury to these very small and precise structures. Twenty pounds for the internal rotation is the maximum I use to avoid injury. As a reminder, I have been doing these exercises for years and I work up to 20 pounds during the peak phase after four months of base and building phases. I use much lighter weights during base and building phases.

Rotator Cuff Internal Rotation

Lying on your side on a bench with a dumbbell in the down hand and a 90 degree bend in your elbow, start with your forearm parallel to the ground and rotate your arm at the shoulder, bringing your hand toward your body. Keep your elbow close to your hip. When lowering the weight to the starting position, make sure your arm does not go past parallel to the ground, as this over-rotation can cause issues.

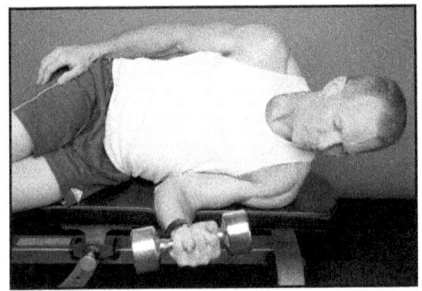 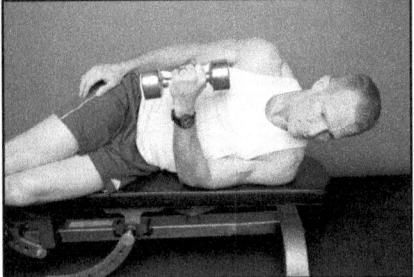

Start — Finish

Rotator Cuff External Rotation

Lying on your side on a bench with a dumbbell in the up hand and a 90-degree bend in your elbow, keep your elbow close to your hip and rotate your forearm away from your body. Before starting this exercise, it is a good idea to place a folded towel between your "up" elbow and body to support your arm. I use about half the weight for external rotation as I do for internal rotation.

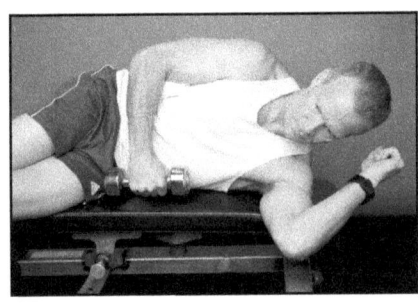 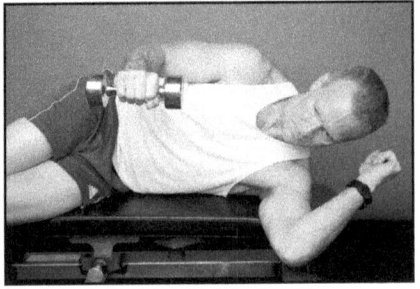

Start — Finish

Rotator Cuff Horizontal Internal Rotation

Lying on your back with a folded towel under your active elbow for support and a lightweight dumbbell in your hand, your upper arm should be perpendicular to your body, with a 90-degree bend in your elbow. Start with the weight near your head and rotate your arm at the shoulder until your hand is directly over your elbow.

Strength Training

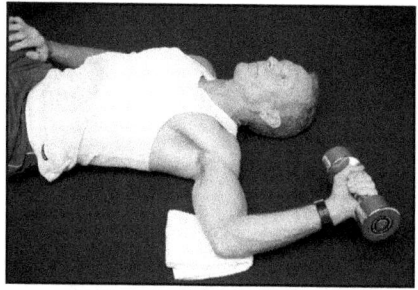 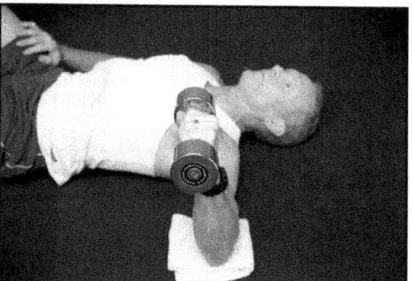

Start — Finish

Rotator Cuff Horizontal External Rotation

Lying on your back with a folded towel under your active elbow for support and a lightweight dumbbell in your hand, your upper arm should be perpendicular to your body, with a 90-degree bend in your elbow. Start with the weight in your hand, directly over your elbow. The start position in this exercise is the same as the finish position for the Horizontal Rotator Cuff Internal Rotation. Rotating at your shoulder, lower the weight so it is near your hip. Depending on flexibility and joint mobility, you may not be able to lower the weight all the way to the floor. If this is the case, lower the weight slowly to your limitation point and let it rest there for a moment, as this will help increase mobility. I use about half the weight for this exercise as I do for the Internal Rotation. As with any of these exercises, if you experience pain, stop and consult a physician.

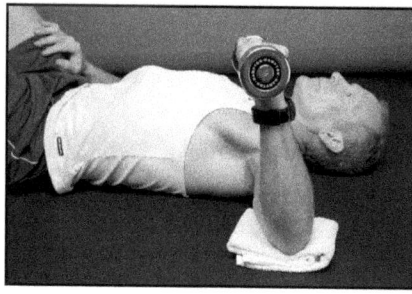 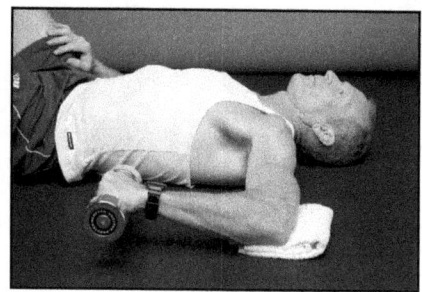

Start — Finish

FRONT DELTOID RAISES

Standing with a dumbbell in each hand and keeping your arms as straight as possible, rotate at the shoulder and raise your hand in front of you to shoulder height. Alternate hands.

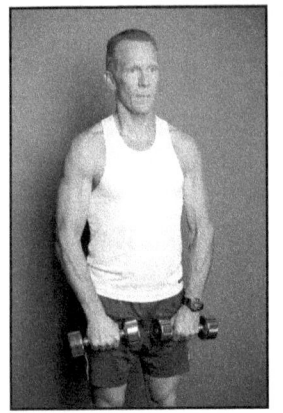
Start

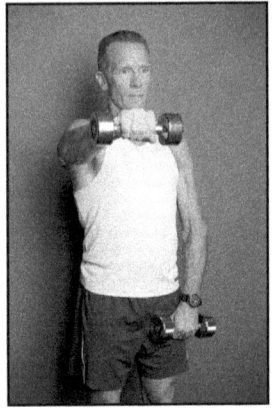
Finish

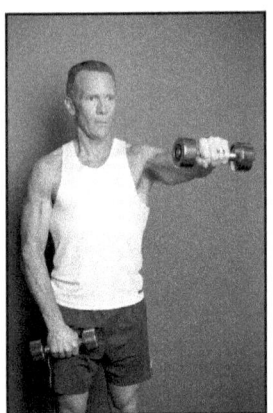
Finish

SIDE DELTOID RAISES

Standing with a dumbbell in each hand and keeping your arms as straight as possible, rotate at the shoulder and raise your hands to the side to shoulder height. To avoid shoulder impingement, make sure your thumbs are pointed up when you reach the top of the movement.

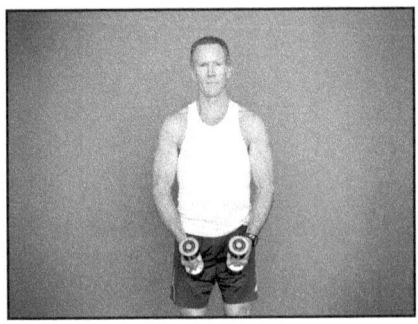
Start

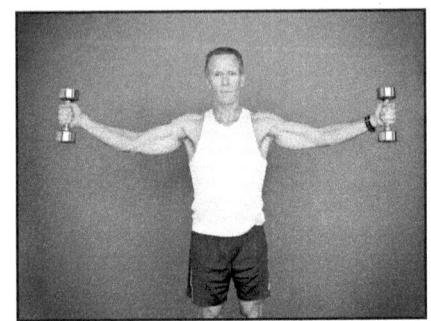
Finish

CORE

Most people don't realize how important the core is. I don't talk about "abs," because to focus on only the abdominal muscles would lead to imbalance and increase the risk of injury. I refer to core work, which refers to abs and lower back muscles, which are above and attach to the pelvis. These need to be strong and flexible to promote a balanced structure, since you will have strong muscles in your legs pulling on the bottom of the pelvis. With proper muscle tension on the front, back, top, and bottom of the pelvis, you create a strong structure against which many very strong and important muscles will pull. This promotes the best structure and mobility possible.

Lower back pain can often be traced to an imbalance in strength or flexibility. In many cases, neglected and weak hamstrings lead to lower back pain and even injury. Many people have stronger quadriceps than any other muscles which attach to the pelvis. Strong quadriceps pull down on the front of the pelvis. If your hamstrings and core are not strong and able to balance the tension created by the quadriceps, this can result in a mild rotation in the pelvis, causing pain in the lower back.

The core exercises in this book may look less rigorous than many abdominal and lower back exercises you may be familiar with, and they are. But they really are all you need to do to have a strong, functional core.

Also, many people think they need to do extensive abdominal workouts to have "six-pack" abs. The truth is, having six-pack abs is more a function of body composition than doing high repetitions of high-resistance abdominal exercises. Most of us have shapely abdominal muscles, but they are hidden by a layer of fat. If you never get rid of this layer of fat, you will never see the six-pack. Smart core and eating programs will produce a great-looking set of abs by creating good muscle tone while also draining the fat away from the abdominal region so they can be seen.

So again, this portion of the strength-training program will help you move better by creating a stronger and more functional core. With regard to weight loss, it is not possible to "spot reduce." That is to say, you cannot target to lose fat in one area of your body. Fat is typically gained or lost throughout the entire body, but various parts of the body gain and lose weight faster than others. For women, the first places they tend to gain and lose fat are the butt and upper legs, while for men it tends to be the belly. Also, when you gain and lose fat it happens near the surface as well as in between and inside muscles. Surface fat is what keeps muscles from looking defined. When I lost 10 pounds a few years ago, the definition of my muscles increased substantially. Logically, I also lost intramuscular fat (fat which is inside muscles) too, which should have made some muscles a little smaller. However, people in the gym asked me if I had put muscle on. This was a result of the optical illusion created by draining much of the fat from my body, which allowed the space between the muscle groups at the surface to be seen more easily.

So, there are a lot of reasons to reduce body fat. Not only will toned abdominal muscles begin to show through; you will gain definition over your entire body. Couple this with the fact that an improved body composition will make you healthier and greatly reduce your risk of contracting the multitude of diseases associated with being "overweight," and losing extra weight should be an easy decision.

CORE EXERCISES

DEAD BUG

Lying on your back with arms extended over your head, bring one arm so it is straight up in the air, and raise the opposite leg with your knee bent at 90 degrees at the same time. As you lower that opposing arm and leg combination, raise the other arm and leg combination. This alternating motion is one of best for activating most of the abdominal and oblique (on the side of your torso) muscles. When doing this exercise for the first time, use only the weight of your arms and legs. Then, after a few weeks, hold a one-pound weight in each hand and place a one-pound weight on each ankle. As it becomes easy at a given weight, increase the weight on each limb. In the most advanced version, keep your legs straight throughout the exercise. Do sets of 20 repetitions.

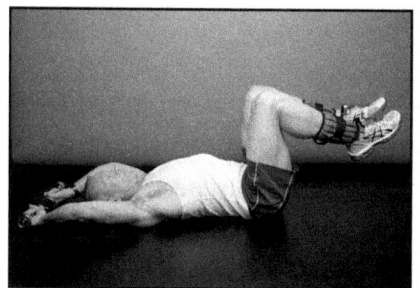 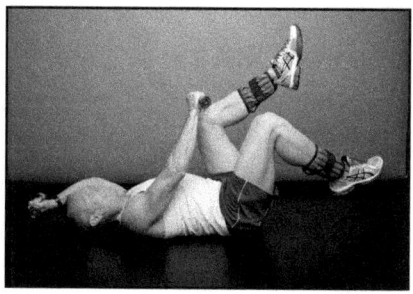

Photos by: Felicity Murphy

Start   Finish

BIRD-DOG

Starting on your hands and knees and keeping your back straight, extend one arm in front of you and the opposing leg behind you. Return to the starting position and alternate.

A more advanced form uses ankle weights and dumbbells. With a dumbbell in your hand, instead of extending an arm in front of you, keep a 90 degree bend in your elbow and raise your arm to your side while extending the opposite leg behind you. Hold for five seconds for five repetitions. As you become stronger, increase the repetitions and holding time until you can do sets of 10 with 10-second holds.

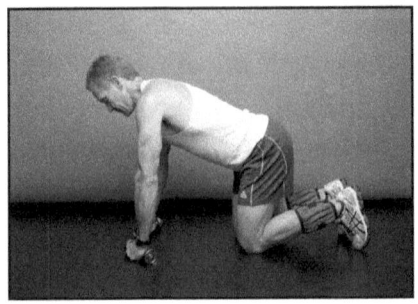 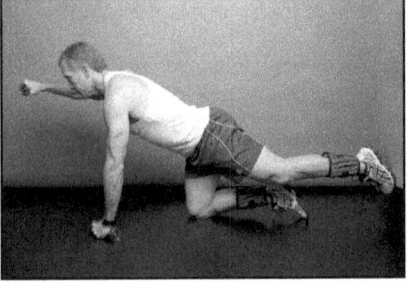

Start   Finish

HOLDING CRUNCH

Lying on your back with your lower back pressed to the floor and your knees bent, place your arms along the side of your body. By contracting your abdominal muscles, raise your head and shoulder blades slightly off the ground and hold. Don't tilt your head forward, as this is bad for your spine. Be sure to keep your spine in proper alignment by keeping your head in the same position relative to your shoulders when you are standing straight up. Do 5 repetitions, and as you get stronger add repetitions and holding time until you are doing 10 reps with 10-second holds.

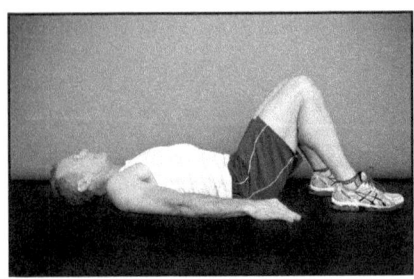 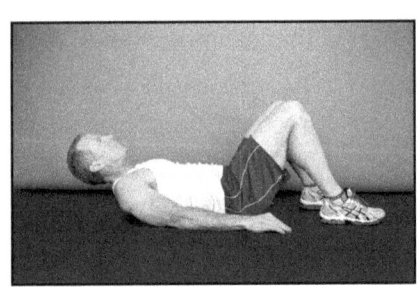

Start   Finish

THE BRIDGE

Start by lying down on your back with your arms at your sides, palms down, with knees bent and feet flat on the floor. Keeping your hands on the floor, raise your pelvis off the floor until your knees, hips and shoulders are in a straight line and hold for 5 seconds. Do 5 repetitions, and as you get stronger, add repetitions and holding time until you are doing 10 reps with 10-second holds. For the advanced version, alternate extending a leg during each 10-count. This exercise works the entire core as well as your gluteals and hamstrings.

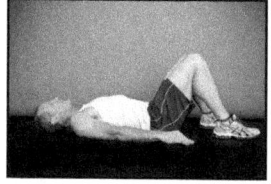 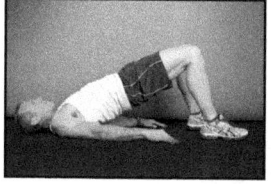 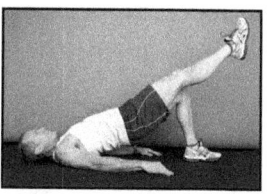

Start   Finish   Advanced

BACK

PULL-DOWNS

Seated on a lat pull-down machine with your upper legs or knees secure under the pad, grasp the bar or handles with a wide grip and pull down so your hands finish close to your shoulders. If using a bar, never pull down so it finishes behind your head.

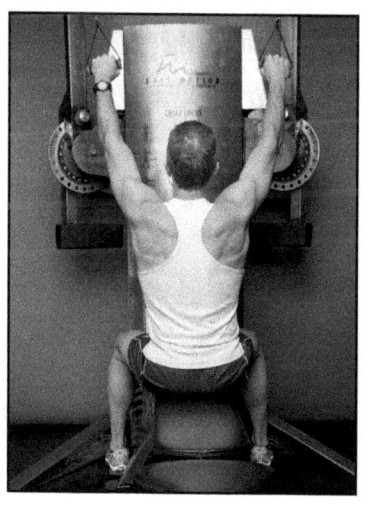 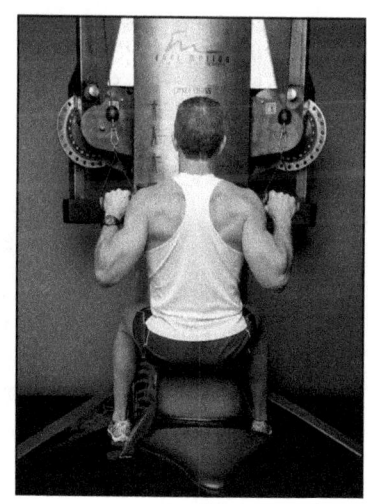

Start   Finish

Seated High Rows

Seated on the cable row machine with feet shoulder-width apart, grasp the bar or handles so they are wider than your shoulders. Pull the bar toward you and finish with your hands near your shoulders. During this movement, keep your back straight and keep your torso in the same position, so you don't rock when starting or finishing the movement.

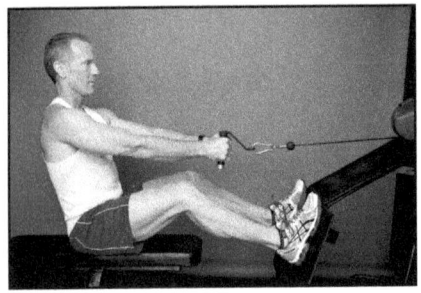 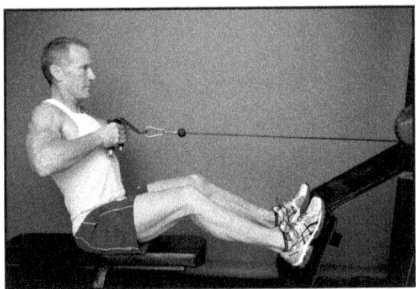

Start | Finish

Dumbbell Pull-over

Lying face up on a bench, start by extending a dumbbell, using both hands, directly over your chest. Rotating at the shoulder, and keeping your arms straight, lower the weight so your arms are parallel to the floor, and then return to the start position.

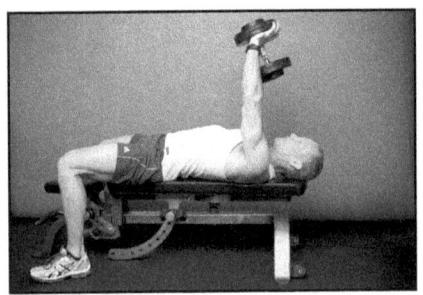 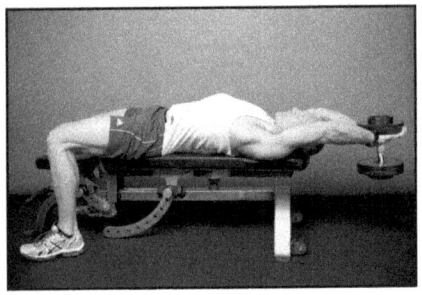

Start | Finish

ONE-ARM DUMBBELL ROW

With the left arm and knee on a bench, grasp the dumbbell with your right hand, set your shoulder, and pull the weight up, finishing with it close to your hip. You already hit the upper part of your lats with the Seated High Row exercise. The One Arm Dumbbell Row works the lower portion of the muscle group by finishing near your hip.

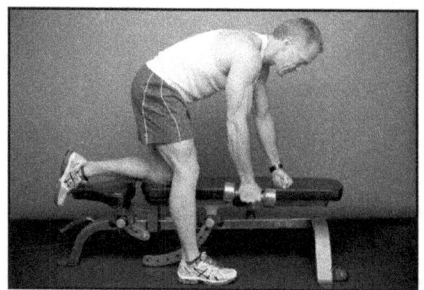 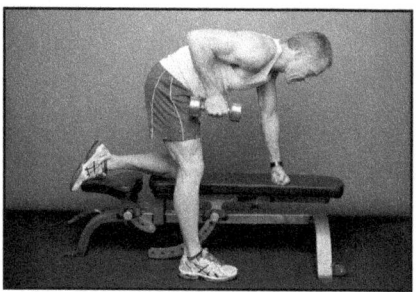

Start   Finish

CHEST

DUMBBELL FLAT BENCH PRESS

Lying on your back on a flat bench, press the weights up, until your arms are fully extended. Lower the weights so they are near your shoulders and your upper arms are parallel to the floor. Taking this exercise deeper than parallel to the floor can lead to shoulder issues.

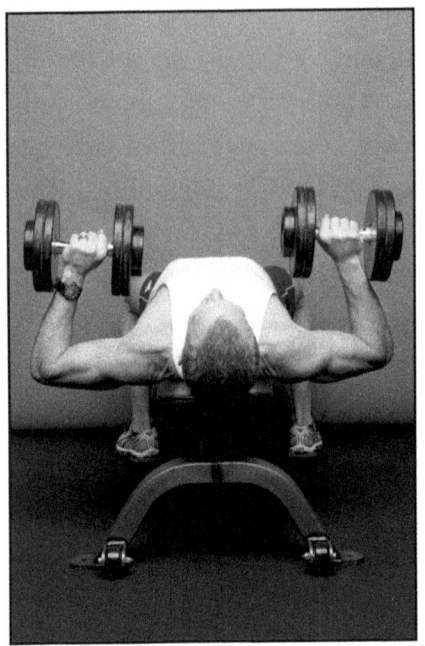 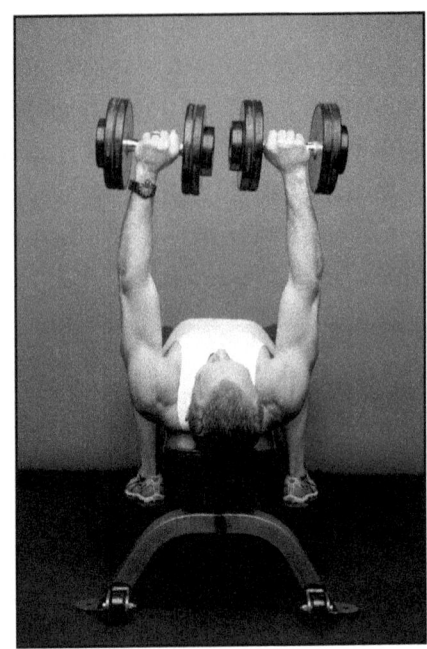

Start   Finish

DUMBBELL FLAT BENCH FLIES

Lying on your back on a flat bench with the dumbbells at your chest, press the weights up, until your arms are fully extended. You are now ready to begin the fly movement. Keeping your arms as straight as possible, rotate out at the shoulder, lowering the weights so your upper arms are parallel to the ground. Old-school technique would have you take the weights way past parallel to get the full "range of motion." More recent evidence indicates that taking this movement past parallel leads to injury. Accordingly, take this movement only as deep as parallel. At the finish position of this exercise, your hands will be only a few inches wider than the "start" position of the Dumbbell Flat Bench Press.

Strength Training

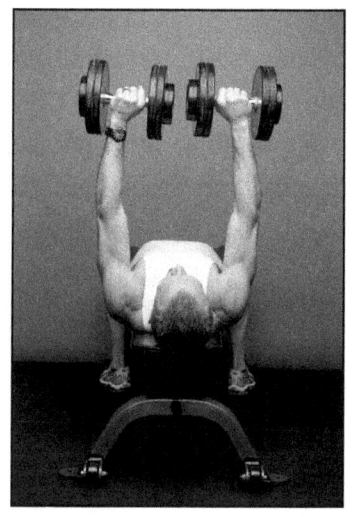

Start

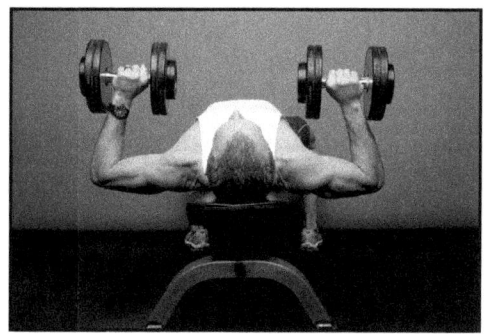

Finish

Dumbbell Incline Bench Press

Lying on your back on an incline bench, bring the dumbbells to your chest. With the back of your hands facing your shoulders, press the weights straight up, until your arms are fully extended.

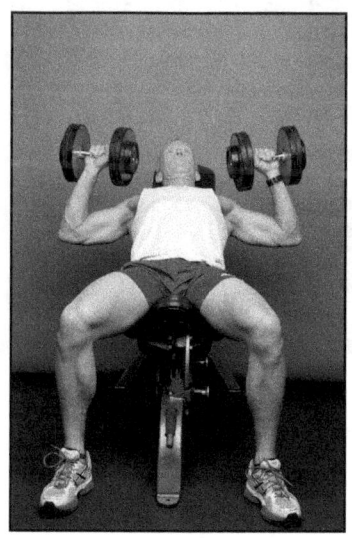

Start

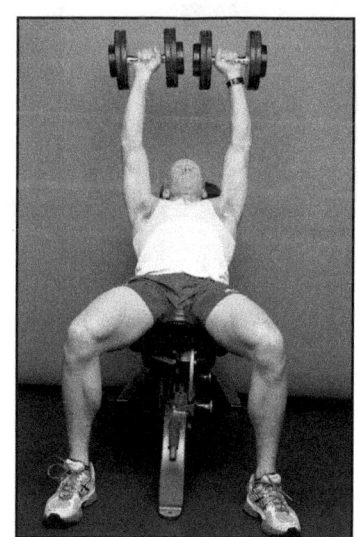

Finish

DUMBBELL INCLINE BENCH FLIES

Lying on your back on a bench, bring the dumbbells to your chest and then press them up so they are directly over your shoulders. Keeping your arms as straight as possible and rotating at the shoulder, lower the weights to the side so your upper arms are parallel to the ground. At the finishing position of this exercise, your hands will be just a few inches wider than at the finish of the Dumbbell Incline Bench Press.

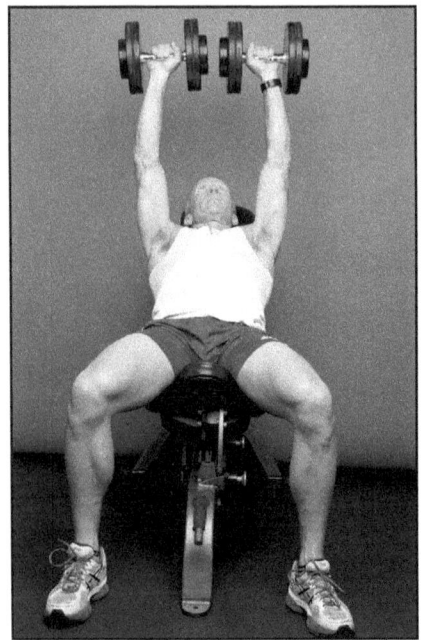

Start

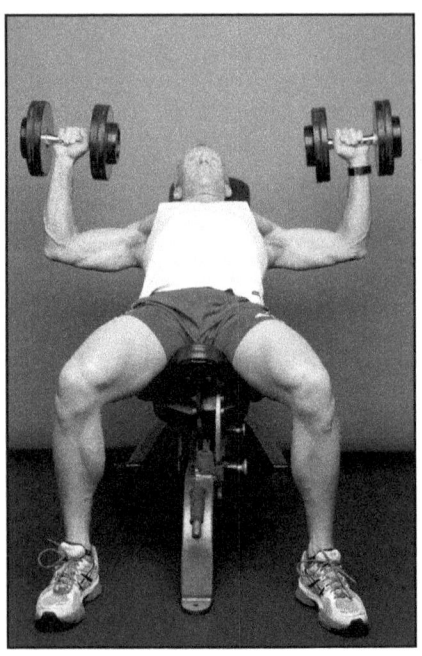

Finish

Cable Decline Press

On a dual cable machine, with the pullies set in a high position, grasp a handle with each hand, and bring the handles to the sides of your chest. Take one or two steps forward, and lean forward so you can press the handles at about a 45-degree angle toward the floor.

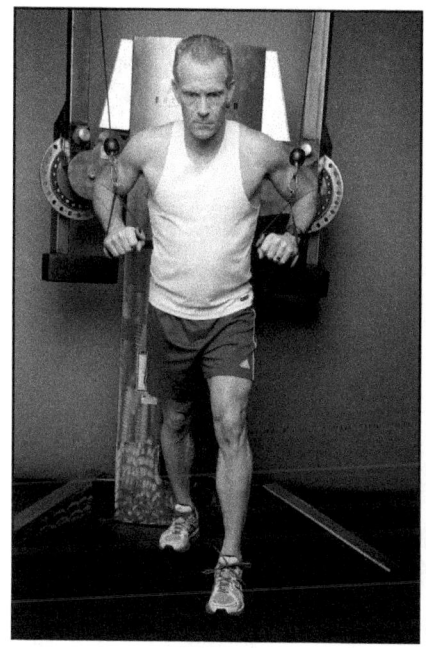

Start

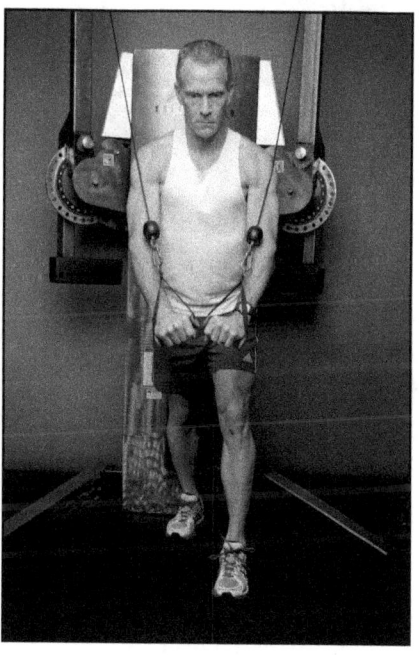

Finish

CABLE DECLINE FLIES

On a dual cable machine, with the pullies set in a high position, grasp a handle with each hand, and bring the handles to the sides of your chest. Press each handle on about a 45-degree angle toward the floor. Then, keeping your arms as straight as possible, rotate your arms at your shoulders to the side until your hands are roughly in line with your shoulders. To finish the movement, rotate your arms back down to the start position.

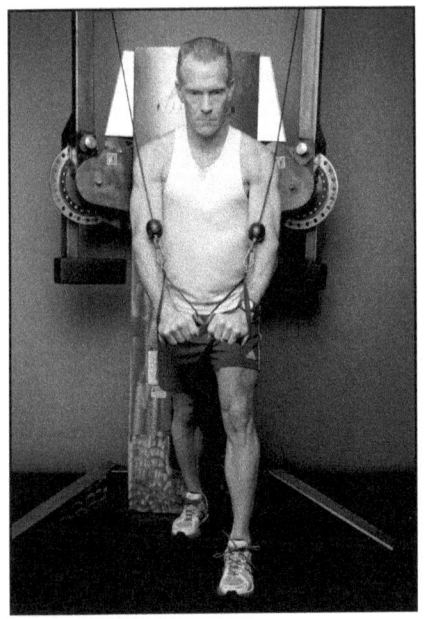
Start

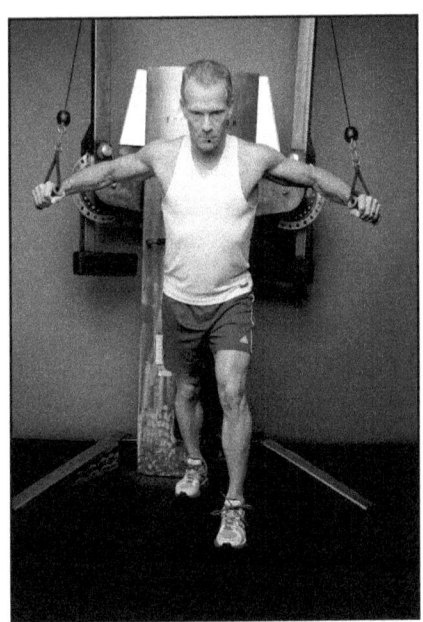
Finish

ARMS

CABLE BICEP CURLS

I like to start my arm routine on a cable machine and super-set them with tricep extensions. To do this, stand up straight, with straight arms at your sides and a handle in each hand with palms facing away from you. Bend your arms at the elbows, and bring the handles to your chest.

Strength Training

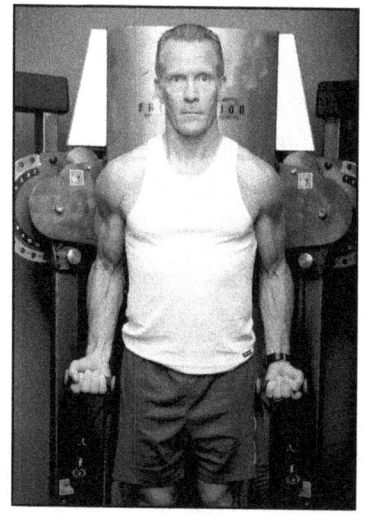
Start

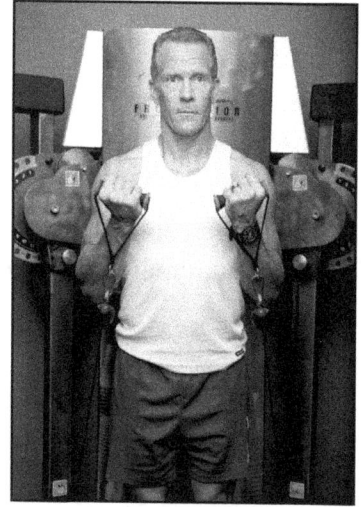
Finish

Cable Tricep Extensions

Standing straight, with bent arms and the handles or rope in your hands, press down until your arms are straight.

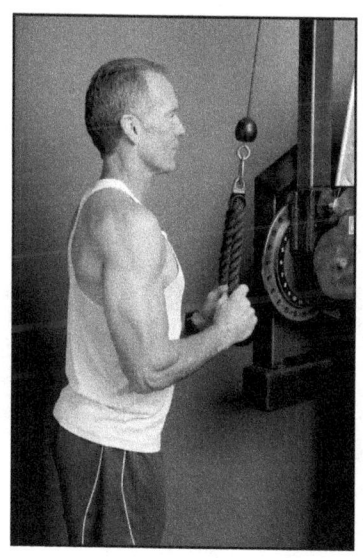
Start

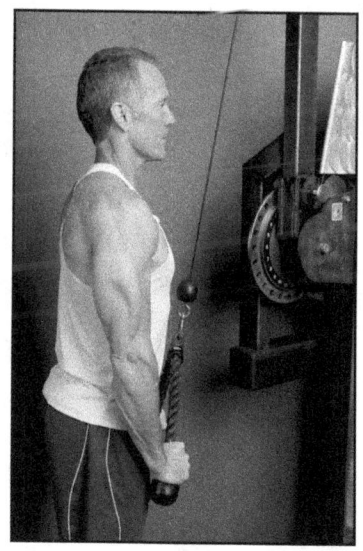
Finish

KICK-BACK TRICEP EXTENSIONS

You can do this exercise with both arms at the same time by bending forward at the waist so your torso is parallel to the ground, while keeping your back straight. However, I prefer to do this exercise on a bench in order to provide lower back support, and do one arm at a time. With one hand and one knee on a bench and a dumbbell in the other hand, pull your arm up so your elbow is at your hip with your lower arm pointing down. Rotate at the elbow and extend your arm back so it is as straight and parallel to the ground as possible.

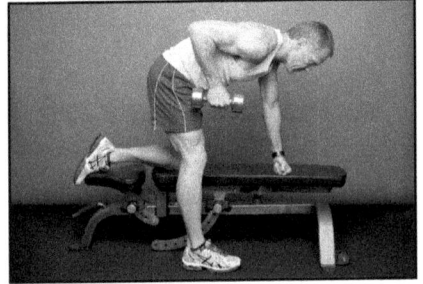
Start

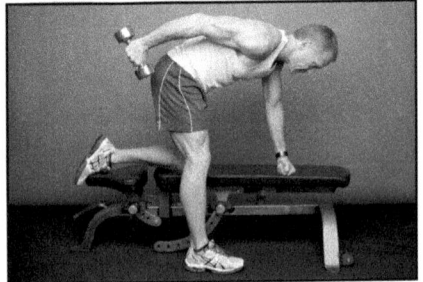
Finish

FINGERTIP FOREARM BARBELL OR DUMBBELL CURLS

With a barbell or dumbbells in your hands, sit on a bench and place the back of your forearms on top of your legs, palms up with your wrists over your knees. With the barbell or dumbbells resting in between the first and second knuckles, close your hand and rotate at the wrist, pulling the weight as high as possible.

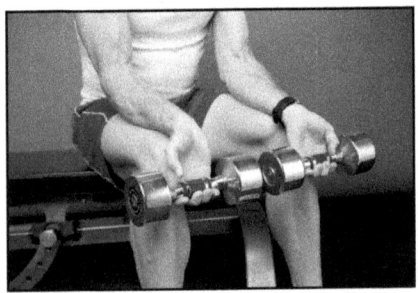
Start

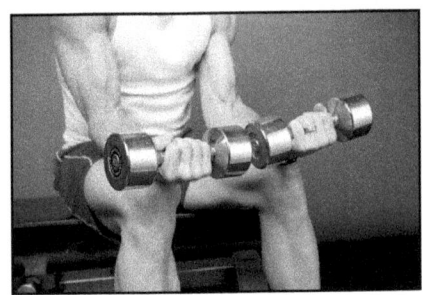
Finish

Strength Training

Seated Reverse Forearm Dumbbell Curls

With dumbbells in your hands, sit on a bench, placing your forearms on your legs with your palms facing down. With your wrists slightly past your knees, rotate at the wrist and raise the weight as high as possible.

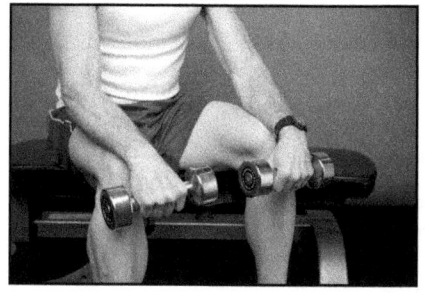
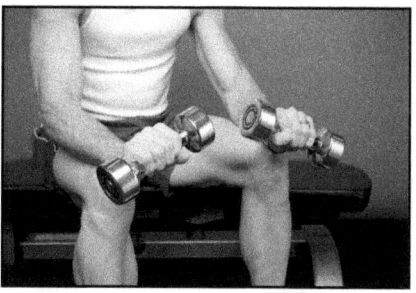

Start   Finish

21s (Reverse Forearm Barbell or Dumbbell Curls)

This is a three-part exercise, with each part performed in sequence without stopping. Standing with a barbell or dumbbells in your hands, with palms facing down and with straight arms, start by bending at the elbow until your forearms are parallel with the ground. Do seven repetitions and then bring the weight all the way to your upper chest, and then lower it until the forearms are again parallel with the ground. Do seven repetitions and then lower your forearms so the weight is all the way in the down position; then bring the weight from the down position to your upper chest and do seven more repetitions, for a total of 21. In base phase, lower the weight and do a few more repetitions.

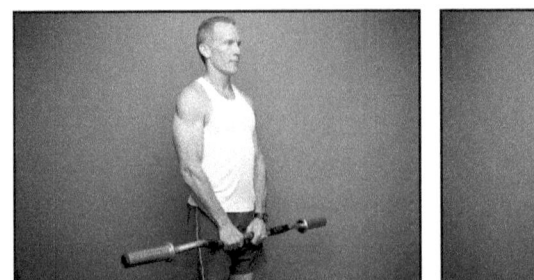
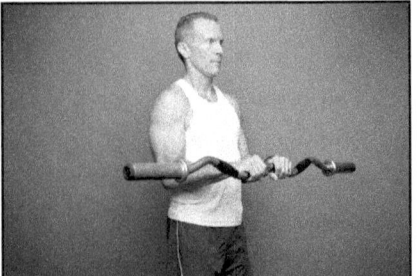

Start Finish

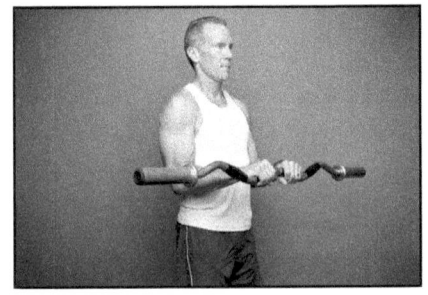
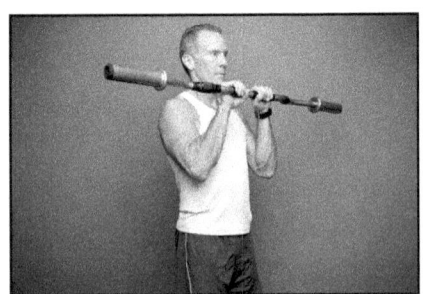

Start Finish

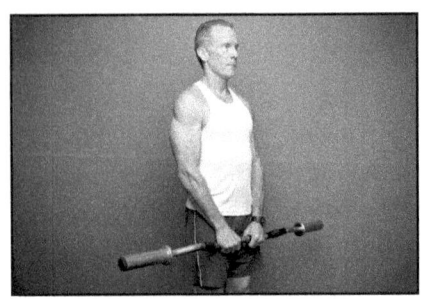
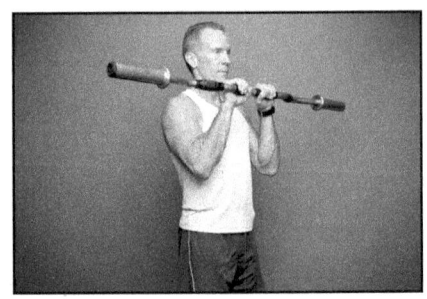

Start Finish

15. Hydration

AN EXTREMELY IMPORTANT COMPONENT OF JUST ABOUT EVERY function that takes place within us is water. Water is the major part of our saliva, stool, and urine, and it also cushions and lubricates brain and joint tissue. It transports nutrients to and carries waste from cells, and it helps regulate body temperature by distributing heat and cooling the body through perspiration. So, it's really important to stay properly hydrated for everyday activities and when you exercise.

During everyday activities, the average person loses two to three quarts of water through breathing and perspiring, and through kidney and intestine function. A quart is 32 fluid ounces. The key to staying hydrated is to take in as much fluid as you lose, but that does not mean you need to drink two to three quarts of water to do it.

Many of the foods we eat, like us, are composed primarily of water. So, if we eat foods that have a high water content we need to figure out how much water, or other fluids which contain water, we need to drink to stay hydrated. I have a simple way to determine if you are hydrated, and we will use the color of your urine as a gauge. I will discuss this further in a moment.

First, let's talk about foods and beverages that can help us stay hydrated. Foods particularly high in water content include most fruits and vegetables. Caffeinated beverages such as soft drinks, tea, and coffee have gotten a bad rap in recent years, and a common misconception has emerged: that such drinks will dehydrate you. Dehydration occurs when you lose more fluid than you take in. More recent information suggests that many caffeinated beverages do have some hydration value.

This notion is contrary to the previously and widely accepted belief that caffeinated beverages have a diuretic effect. According to Katherine Zeratsky, R.D., L.D., Mayo Clinic Nutritionist, researchers used to believe that caffeinated beverages had a diuretic effect. This means that you would urinate more after drinking them, which could increase the risk of becoming dehydrated. Recent research shows that this is not true and that caffeine has a diuretic effect only if consumed in large amounts, more than 500 to 600 milligrams, or the equivalent of five to seven cups of coffee a day. This means I will continue to have my one strong cup of coffee every morning.

I am not trying to suggest you drink only caffeinated beverages to stay hydrated. I am simply trying to clarify information that is widely accepted in society, but is wrong. I do this so that if a caffeinated beverage is one of your favorite "foods," you can continue to enjoy it, without feeling like you are doing something wrong.

The old anecdotal formula for proper hydration was: 8 glasses of 8 fluid ounces of water a day, for a total of 64 ounces. If you drink that amount of water and still have food and other beverages that have hydration value, you could become a little overhydrated. To clarify, it is better to be a little overhydrated than to be a little underhydrated. The question then becomes: how do you know if you are either?

The old anecdotal rule that indicated proper hydration was to keep drinking water until your urine is clear. The belief was that if very dark urine is a sign of dehydration, clear urine must mean you are properly hydrated. However, completely clear urine usually means your body has plenty of water, and should serve to indicate you are well-hydrated. Conversely, dark urine is an indication of being underhydrated and can indicate that you are dehydrated. Dark urine means you are low on fluids and your urine is condensed, so the electrolyte molecules, which make the color of your urine, are

HYDRATION

closer than they should be. It is also important to note that dark urine can also be caused by certain foods, vitamins, and medications; so, if your urine is dark, it could be the onset of dehydration if the other possible causes are not present.

My own general physician, an internal medicine specialist, agrees with a growing number of other experts, that a good anecdotal way to know you are properly hydrated is to keep an eye on the color of your urine. When you are properly hydrated, your urine will be a light yellow. This does not mean you can't drink any more water that day; it just means you should drink additional fluids based on your thirst, for everyday activities.

I like using urine color as a hydration guide because it is simple. Rather than trying to measure the exact amount of fluids I have lost and then need to replace, I can simply monitor my urine and have a pretty good idea of my hydration and make changes as needed. The simplicity of monitoring my hydration is similar to the simplicity of my system of monitoring my caloric balance through the use of a scale. Rather than calculate every calorie I consume and burn, I can simply weigh myself every day to see where I am. If I am a little up or a little down in weight, I can usually identify the cause from the previous day and then adjust as necessary. Since I can keep track of where I am and make adjustments to stay close to where I want to be, I don't get stressed out about my weight, because I am in control of it. It's also a good idea to start every day with at least a 12-ounce glass of water to replace the fluid loss from breathing while you were sleeping.

Proper exercise hydration is very different from non-exercise hydration, and it starts the night before. If you are going to exercise or race the next morning, drink 16 ounces of a caffeine-free beverage before bed. In the morning, start the day with another 16 ounces of caffeine-free beverage. I prefer a sports drink, which has some carbohydrates, protein, and electrolytes. Since I exercise most mornings, I have found this to rehydrate me and give me some fuel for the workout.

During high-exertion workouts or races, drink four to eight ounces every fifteen minutes by taking several big gulps. Larger gulps help trigger the absorption process better than sipping. Also, if using a sports drink instead of gels during high exertions, the drink should contain carbohydrates and protein in a ratio of 4:1. A recent study determined the addition of this ratio of carbohydrate to protein extended endurance by 57% over water alone, and 24% over a carbohydrate-only drink. When the drink also included electrolytes, such as sodium and potassium, not only did the performance improve during the activity by replenishing electrolytes lost in respiration and perspiration, it also enhanced recovery.

Exercise Nutrition

The human body uses three types of fuel for energy: carbohydrate, fat and protein. The level and duration of exertion determines which fuel, or combination of fuel sources are used. During lower level exertions, fat is the primary fuel while during higher level exertions it shifts to carbohydrate. During longer and higher exertions 5 to 15% of your energy can come from protein.

Recently consumed carbohydrate, called glucose, will remain in the blood stream and will be used first during exercise. Carbohydrate stored in the liver and muscles is called glycogen. The average person can store about 2000 calories of glycogen and about 80,000 calories in fat. Stored protein is muscle tissue itself.

Since most of us have relatively large fat stores, there is no need to put fat into your blood stream during exercise. This will force the body to take it from fat stores. Carbohydrates and protein are a different story. During higher exertions it is better to consume these so they are taken directly from the blood stream, thus protecting stored glycogen and protein.

Protecting glycogen is less important than protecting stored protein, since stored protein refers to muscle tissue. If protein is not present in the blood stream the body will take what it needs from existing muscle tissue: essentially cannibalizing itself. By taking protein from existing muscle tissue, muscle damage is increased adding to the damage done to muscles through micro-tears during normal exercise. This additional damage can dramatically increase the amount of time needed for muscles to repair themselves.

The good news is: this can easily be prevented through proper nutrition during exercise, especially higher and longer exertions. By consuming a drink or gel with a carbohydrate to protein ratio of 4 to 1 during higher and longer exertions, you allow the body to use glucose and protein in the bloodstream as fuel, protecting stores and dramatically reducing muscle damage and recovery time.

16. Post-Workout and Race Nutrition

A WASTED WORKOUT IS ONE WHICH IS NOT IMMEDIATELY FOL-lowed with proper nutrition. When you finish a workout or race, you have a window of about 30 minutes to give the muscles what they need to begin the healing and replenishing process, which is also known as recovery. Studies show that when you optimize the recovery process through proper nutrition and rest, you maximize the adaptation process by allowing muscles to heal faster and more completely.

During exercise, glycogen stores can be depleted, which must then be replenished. For about 30 minutes following a workout or race, muscle cells are dilated and are ready to absorb fluids and glucose, which will replenish glycogen stores. Also, protein is needed in the blood stream to begin the repair process of normal cell damage caused by micro-tears during exercise. If protein is not present in the bloodstream in this 30-minute window, the body will cannibalize other undamaged muscle tissue to obtain it, increasing muscle damage and lengthening the time needed to repair it.

Proper post-workout or race nutrition, coupled with the right kind of rest, promotes the fastest and most complete recovery possible. When you recover better, you can exert at a higher level again sooner. This is most important during peak-phase workouts, since these will involve the highest intensity. For example, the more completely you recover from a Tuesday track workout, the more you will be able to exert at a higher level, and more easily, during a Thursday hill run. Being able to exert at a higher level during these workouts will maximize the adaptation response, resulting in greater improvements in strength and speed.

The penalty for missing this 30-minute window is that your muscles won't get what they need and additional damage will occur as the muscles take protein from existing muscles to repair the micro-tears caused by the exercise. This will dramatically hamper the recovery process.

When I started training the right way 10 years ago, I started drinking Endurox R-4 immediately following a workout or race. It has the 4:1 carbohydrate to protein ratio, which is now widely accepted as the appropriate ratio to optimize the recovery process. Since then, before every workout I put two scoops in a drink bottle and put that in my gym bag. As soon as the workout is over, I add 12 ounces of water and drink it immediately. A number of weight-conscious people I have coached have been concerned that the carbohydrates in this post workout drink will cause weight gain. The only time this should be a concern is during the base phase. Low-intensity exertions for less than an hour may not cause a significant amount of muscle damage and may not deplete glycogen stores in a significant way. So, for low-intensity workouts that last less than one hour, recovery requirements may be different. However, I have a recovery drink after every workout.

This means that, by following a higher-intensity workout with a proper recovery drink, you will recover better and faster and make the muscles stronger. This process, if coupled with a smart eating program, will lead to an increase in lean muscle mass and a reduction in stored fat.

17. Eating Program

THIS EATING PROGRAM IS ONE OF THE KEYS TO BECOMING MORE healthy and fit. It is not a diet. A diet is something you do for a short period of time and requires being deprived of many, if not all, of your favorite foods. This program is not a diet, because it is the way you should eat for the rest of your life, and it includes eating many, if not all, of your favorite foods.

Four years ago, during a vacation up the coast, my wife took a picture of me coming out of the ocean. I was fit but fat. Everything was just a little looser than I cared for, so I decided I would lose some weight. I did some research and then used the following eating program to lose about 10 pounds, and I did it without changing the volume or intensity of my workouts. It was easy to do because this eating program is about moderation, not deprivation.

The first physical I had following my weight loss led to a conversation with my doctor out of concern for a medical issue. After explaining that I had intended to lose the weight, and that I had lost it using a safe program, she explained a study she had read in the New England Journal of Medicine which looked at four different weight loss programs. One focused on reducing carbohydrates, another on reducing fat, and the others focused on reducing other foods. The conclusion of the study was that it didn't matter if you reduced carbohydrates or fat, the key was to reduce calories. I prefer my eating program because it focuses on putting the right calories in the right amounts in the right parts of the day, while still allowing me to eat all of my favorite foods.

When I started training for sprint triathlons, I increased the number of cardiovascular workouts I did each week. This caused me to burn a lot more calories, and I began to lose more weight. I used this as an opportunity to find my strength balance point relative to my weight. At 165 pounds I was fine, but when I got down to 163 I noticed my strength began to suffer. To solve this problem, I put the weight back on by eating more carbohydrates at night. It took about two weeks to get back to 165, and my strength returned. This became my new balance point and is my race weight today. It's also what I weighed in college.

If I had to pick a single modification to spur weight loss, I would recommend the elimination of carbohydrates after 6:00 p.m. That's because most of us aren't that active after 6:00 p.m., so carbohydrates we eat after that will only be stored as fat while we sleep. If most people implement only this part of the eating program, they can lose weight. However, to achieve proper nutritional balance, better energy, and improved health, I recommend you consult a physician and then use the entire program, especially since it is so easy to follow.

This program does not require you to know and think about every gram of carbohydrates, protein, and fat you eat, but you do need to be aware of a few numbers as guidelines. I find trying to be too precise about the exact amount of each of these food groups in each meal is very difficult. The stress and frustration caused by programs which call for very precise measurements in every meal make such programs very difficult to follow consistently, and this is why people can't stay on them.

When we think of moderation and not deprivation, this means indulging now and then. For example, if you are watching your fat intake and you normally eat lean meat, and are losing the weight you want to, you can have a rib-eye steak now and again, if that is what you want. The key is to indulge within reason and without guilt. If you follow the program most of the time and are seeing the results you want, indulging once in a while will be a reward that will help you stay on the program long-term.

This program requires a little homework up front, so you know the actual value of what you are eating, and to establish a baseline. By determining the composition of the foods you eat every day, you will be able to identify areas you need to change to achieve your goals.

This program also involves weighing yourself, so you will need to buy an accurate scale. Many people are averse to the use of scales. Many women I know never get on a scale, and they recoil at the thought of getting one. In fairness, they monitor their weight by gauging how their clothes fit. If a certain pair of pants is a little "snug," they know they need to lose a few pounds.

However, I prefer to use actual numbers on the scale to see where I am. If I am up a few pounds, I can usually look back over the previous several days and identify what I ate or drank to cause the weight gain. A scale is just telling the truth. The aversion many have to getting on a scale is because the scale does tell the truth. I say, embrace the truth. Don't obsess over it, but use the information to better understand what your body is doing to better fine-tune your eating road map to success.

Nutritionists recommend you consume on a daily basis 50 to 60% of your calories from carbohydrates like fruits, vegetables, and whole grains; 15 to 25% from protein like cottage cheese, eggs, chicken, fish, beef, or soy; and 20 to 25% from fat like olives, avocados, nuts or seeds. That's right: fat, of the right kind and in the right amount, actually helps certain bodily functions.

The Harvard School of Public Health says, "The total amount of fat you eat, whether high or low, isn't really linked with disease. What really matters is the *type of fat* you eat.

The "bad" fats—saturated and trans fats—increase the risk for certain diseases. The "good" fats—monounsaturated and polyunsaturated fats—lower disease risk. The key to a healthy diet is to substitute good fats for bad fats—and to avoid trans fats.

Although it is still important to limit the amount of cholesterol you eat, especially if you have diabetes, dietary cholesterol isn't nearly the villain it's been portrayed to be. Cholesterol in the bloodstream is what's most important. And the biggest influence on blood cholesterol level is the mix of fats in your diet—not the amount of cholesterol you eat from food. To identify the fat content and type of fat in foods, read the label. In a restaurant, it's good to avoid fried food unless you know the restaurant doesn't use trans fats."

This program provides a general framework, and finding your caloric balance will require a little trial and error. Again, while I am trying to keep it as simple as possible, you should be familiar with a couple of numbers regarding dietary values. There are about 3500 calories in a pound of fat. This means that if you are already in caloric balance -- that is to say, your weight doesn't change much from day to day -- by reducing your daily caloric intake by 500 you will lose a pound of fat in one week. However, if you normally consume a very high number of calories, which puts you way out of caloric balance, reducing 500 a day may not produce any weight loss, but it may slow your weight gain.

It's a simple matter of calories consumed compared to the number of calories burned each day. If you consume 3000 calories a day and only burn 2000 you can reduce your caloric intake by 500 to 2500 and you will still be taking in 500 excess calories a day, which is 3500 a week, and you will gain 1 pound of fat in that week. This is where the scale comes in. Weigh yourself every morning on an accurate scale. If your weight stays the same from week to week, then you are in caloric balance.

For many people who struggle with weight issues, the solution will come by combining a smart exercise program that increases the number of calories burned along with a smart eating program that reduces the number of calories consumed, while still providing all the necessary nutrients. So, if you consume your recommended caloric intake, and burn that number of calories in a day, your weight should not change. You can then increase your activity level or decrease your caloric intake slightly, and in most cases you will safely lose weight.

It sounds simple because it is. The key is modifying your activity level or caloric intake, or both, in ways that are reasonable and sustainable. If you remember, I lost 10 pounds in about three months at age 47 by reducing my caloric intake by cutting my carbohydrate intake, while my activity level remained the same.

If you try this program and make caloric or exercise adjustments and your goal is to lose weight, but you don't, there may be other factors affecting you which cannot be covered in this book. In that case, consult your doctor or certified nutritionist and consider having a test done to determine your Resting Metabolic Rate (RMR). RMR determines exactly how many calories you use to maintain basic life functions like: brain activity, heart and lung function, tissue growth and repair, and internal organ function. If you then calculate how many calories you burn during exercise and combine that number with your RMR, you can determine with great precision how many calories you should consume each day if you want to lose weight.

I prefer the more simple method of identifying my caloric balance by using a scale every day. As a starting point, I also recommend mapping what you eat every day for one week. This will require a little homework up front, but the education you will gain from doing it will pay dividends for the rest of your life, since you will know what the foods you eat contain, and what they do to you. I recommend logging everything you eat for a week and note the number of calories, grams of carbohydrates, protein, and fat, and include the type of fat. I did this recently and it was an eye-opener. I learned that I consume between 3000 and 3500 calories a day, but it turns out that's about right for a guy my size, with my activity level.

EATING PROGRAM

To figure out in general what your caloric intake should be, there are several online tools you can use, like <u>healthycalculators.com</u>. They will ask for your age, height, weight, and activity level to calculate your recommended caloric intake. This is a ballpark estimate of what you should consume each day to maintain your weight. I plugged my numbers in recently and they calculated I should intake around 3100 calories a day, which is about right.

Also keep in mind that exercising is not the only way we burn calories. All of the other things we do in a day cause us to burn calories, from reading the newspaper, to cooking, to interacting with colleagues at work, or running a household. This is why you should not spend too much time trying to calculate the exact number of calories you will burn when you work out to achieve your caloric burn goal.

You should have a general idea that certain activities will burn calories at a certain rate, as well as an idea of how many calories are in the foods you eat. But rather than try to calculate your caloric intake and burn with too much precision each day, simply eat smart and get on a scale every day to map your progress. The concept will take a little getting used to, but in the long term you will have the tools you need to stay in control of the most important thing you have: your health.

You should find that by tracking what you eat for a week, you will discover why you have been gaining weight. By using this information, coupled with the eating program below, you will have the ability to identify foods you are eating too much of and/or at the wrong time of the day. This information will allow you to manage those foods better. There are a number of online tools you can use, like <u>my-calorie-counter.com</u> to help map your caloric intake, as well as identify the carbohydrate, protein, and fat content of almost any food.

Again, you are going to map your food intake and the value of each food for only one week. In the end, the time commitment to do this will be minimal, but it will pay maximum dividends by taking control of how you eat.

In this eating program, again, to keep it simple, I call for portion sizes you can measure without having to weigh anything. For instance, a "handful" of something is often called for. That means the portion you should eat is roughly the amount of that food which fills your open hand. The exact amount will vary from person to person, and you will need to experiment a little to find the amount of food which gets you through to the next meal, but still allows you to lose weight. This is where weighing yourself every day will be very helpful.

I have found that on many Mondays I retain a couple of pounds of fluid from the weekend. I have also found that, if I am good Monday night and don't have any alcohol while watching Monday Night Football, I can lose as much as two pounds by Tuesday morning. As a side note, my research has identified beer and salted buttered popcorn, two of my favorite foods, cause the fluid retention I see on many Monday mornings.

If you want more precise guidance, consult a certified nutritionist. Also, having a conversation with your doctor during your annual physical is a good idea to make sure you are on the right track. If you want meals that are already prepared, there are several companies that offer such meals. I prefer to prepare my own food because it is less expensive and tastes better than pre-made diet meals.

When I started this eating program, I didn't lose any weight for the first two weeks. This was the result of the decrease in calories, which caused my body to go into a "famine" mode. This is when the body reacts to a decrease in calories by slowing the metabolic rate in order to retain fat stores. This is normal. Then, after two weeks, I started losing about half a pound a week. I know this because I was using a very accurate scale at work and I weighed myself each morning prior to working out.

Everyone I have given this eating program to has had the same result. They lose the weight, which improved their overall health. Then, when they added the rest of the program with good stretching, strength training, and some cardiovascular exercise, their overall health improved, giving them better appearance, energy, and confidence.

Perhaps the best part of this program for people like me, who like to have some wine or a beer or two on the weekends, is that you can. Even though these drinks are usually pretty high in calories, if the rest of your week is in balance, you can have a few drinks on the weekend and be fine. Remember, this program is not about deprivation -- it's about moderation and proper balance.

Most people think protein has fewer calories per gram than carbohydrates. This is incorrect. Protein and carbohydrates have the same number of calories per gram, 4, while fat has 9 calories per gram. The down side of protein is that it can contain a lot of fat. The up side of protein is that the body burns more calories digesting it compared to carbohydrates. So, opt for leaner meat, fish, or poultry when possible, but when you want a rib-eye steak on occasion, have the rib-eye and don't feel guilty about it. Occasional indulgence is part of a balanced program, because it makes it easier to stay on the right path.

I also recommend taking a multivitamin every day. No matter how precise you are in trying to get all of the needed nutrients from what you eat, you probably won't. Taking a multivitamin every day ensures you will. Also, multivitamins are gender-specific, since men and women have different nutritional needs, so make sure you get the right one.

Below you will find the eating program. It is a guideline. Think of each meal as a set of recommendations. You will need to experiment and tailor your specific eating program to achieve your goals. Also, if you work out first thing in the morning, the carbohydrates called for earlier in the day will be very helpful. If you exercise later in the day, it will be helpful to move some of the carbohydrates from somewhere else in the program to precede your workouts so you have a fresh fuel supply.

You will also notice that this program is not "three square meals a day." It is many meals a day, but some of them might be thought of as "between-meal snacks." Studies show that more smaller meals result in a more even release of energy throughout the day. More meals also help prevent gorging, which can occur when you eat fewer meals.

Another very important part of any eating program is variety. It is important to mix it up and eat a wide variety of foods, so your meals are something you look forward to, because they taste good. Simplicity and ease of use are also important. I have found Trader Joe's to have a lot of really great-tasting and easy-to-prepare foods, which are also really healthy. I will admit, however, that sometimes I will buy a bucket of chicken from a fast food restaurant and eat that as my protein at lunch for a few days. I get away with that because I know my balance points. Also, as a result of getting a complete physical every year, I know all my markers are doing well. My annual physicals also give me the ability to see changes in my physiology, giving me the ability to notice negative trends and make corrective changes in what I eat.

The eating program detailed below is what I recommend to improve fitness and health, and help you lose weight if that is your goal. Following the eating program, I have listed what I eat during an average week. When reviewing my eating habits, remember that everyone is different, and that only very active people can eat like I do and not gain a lot of weight. I want to underscore the need to check with your doctor when deciding to adopt all or part of this program. Salt is everywhere in our diet, and it can be very dangerous. It can cause high blood pressure, which can lead to heart disease and stroke. I eat pretty high amounts of salt, but through my genetics and activity level, I remain "in balance." Again, see your doctor, get a complete physical and find your balance.

In the starting gate, just before the 2010 Malibu triathlon, my fellow competitors and I were looking out at the cold Pacific on that grey and blustery day, when the guy next to me asked rhetorically in a loud voice, "So why do we do this again?" to which I responded, "So we can eat more of our favorite foods." The group had a good laugh. Truth is -- that is one of the greatest benefits of having a balanced life, which includes smart eating and fitness programs.

THE EATING SCHEDULE

MEAL 1: JUST AFTER GETTING UP

1 serving of oatmeal, preferably steel-cut, or a granola bar or other breakfast cereal, but keep the sugar content low. Add blueberries to your oatmeal; they have antioxidants and anti-inflammatory properties, too. Have a glass of water with it.

MEAL 2: AROUND 9:30 A.M.

1 whole egg and three egg whites. Having one whole egg and then three egg whites gives you all the protein you need for that part of the day, and should hold you until lunch. Also, when eating hard-boiled eggs, you may need to salt them. I use Morton Lite Salt, which has half the sodium of table salt, but also contains potassium chloride, which is good for you. If you get tired of hard-boiled eggs, have an omelet or a breakfast burrito. The light carbs in the tortilla won't hurt anything and the variety will help keep you on track.

MEAL 3: LUNCH, AROUND 11:30 A.M.

One handful of fish, chicken, or lean beef.
One handful of green vegetables or a large salad with an oil and vinegar dressing.

Half a handful of sweet potatoes or brown rice.
A piece of fruit for dessert.

Meal 4: Between 3:00 and 4:00 p.m.
A drink or bar, high in protein.

Meal 5: Dinner
One handful of fish, chicken, or lean beef.
One handful of vegetables, like broccoli, asparagus, or Brussel sprouts, or a large salad with oil and vinegar dressing.
(No carbohydrates from starches in this meal)

Meal 6: Evening snack
Protein drink or roasted nuts, with a sugar-free and caffeine-free soda or water. If you need to watch your salt intake, have unsalted nuts.

What I Eat in a Week at Age 52
Again, I consume 3000 to 3500 calories a day, because that is what I burn every day. I know this because I weigh myself every weekday and I can see any changes, because the scale I use is very accurate. While you should be able to stay on the above eating program because it includes the smart placement and amounts of real food, what I eat and the amount of it should serve as encouragement.

I eat a lot of really good food and still have a few beers, and if you are patient, you will be able to eat more of your favorite foods as your fitness improves. I have found it very easy to stay on this plan because the key is moderation, not deprivation. By eating real foods I like, which also meet all of my nutritional needs, I am now in the best shape of my life, and I look forward to every meal.

Eating Program

PRE-WORKOUT

Driving to work I have a powder drink I mix with 12 ounces of water, which has both carbohydrates and protein, along with a granola bar.

POST-WORKOUT

Two scoops of Tangy Orange Endurox R-4 in 12 ounces of water.

AT DESK AT 8:00

A cup of coffee and two small blueberry scones from Trader Joe's.

MID-MORNING SNACK AT 9:30

One whole egg and three egg whites; or a bacon, egg, sour cream, salsa, and cheese quesadilla; or two eggs, two pieces of bacon, and a piece of French toast. I drink a low-calorie sports drink with this meal to further re-hydrate and top off my electrolytes.

LUNCH

One handful of fish, chicken, or beef; one handful of green vegetables or a large salad; half a handful of brown rice; and a diet soda. For dessert, I have one or two dark chocolate peanut butter cups, again from Trader Joes.

4 P.M. SNACK

A protein shake with around 20 grams of protein, and maybe a bag of chips.

6 P.M. DINNER

One handful of fish, chicken, or beef and one handful of green vegetables or a salad.

8:30 P.M. SNACK

When in weight-loss mode, I eat a handful of nuts. When not in weight-loss mode, I eat one or two handfuls of carbohydrates. Either way I have a sugar-free and caffeine-free soda.

Friday Night

My family and I hit our favorite Mexican restaurant and I have some chips with guacamole, taquitos or a taco, a cheese enchilada, and perhaps a Negro Modelo or two.

Weekend

Pre-workout

Saturday is my long bike day, so I have a bowl of granola cereal, and halfway through my ride I sometimes have a granola bar. Following the ride, I skip the Endurox and get a cup of coffee and some food at the local coffee house with my wife.

Lunch

Not as regimented as my workday lunches. My family and I usually end up at a restaurant, and sometimes it's fast food. Remember, it's not fast food that causes a person to gain weight, it's eating the fast food and then not exercising that causes a person to gain weight. On close examination, many fast food restaurants have pretty healthy options. Yes, many have the 1400-calorie burgers with loads of fat and carbohydrates, but many have relatively healthy options. Most if not all now display the calorie and fat content, allowing you to make good convenient choices on the go.

Mid-afternoon snack between 4:00 and 4:30 PM

Usually some cheese, crackers, and salami with a beer.

Eating Program

DINNER

I will grill chicken or steak, but we often hit another great restaurant. I will enjoy a piece of bread, salad, some good fish, chicken, or beef and a beer or two. Sometimes the entreé is a pasta dish with protein.

AFTER DINNER

At the movies, it's "buttered" popcorn and a diet soda.

AFTER THE MOVIE

It's usually a drink or two with my wife before bed.

I have tailored this eating program over the years and I have maintained my caloric balance, as evidenced by my stable weight. During the holiday season, I usually put on three to five pounds, because I love good food. I will easily lose this before the next race season.

I know the foods I enjoy are in balance with my overall health. This is because I get regular physicals that measure all critical areas. Moving forward, if I fall outside of any of the parameters measured during my physical, I will adjust my eating accordingly. But, for now, I eat all of my favorite foods, and since I eat the right amounts of each, I have the energy to do all of my favorite things too.

18. Starting Your Cardiovascular Program

NOW THAT WE HAVE THE STRETCHING, STRENGTH TRAINING, AND eating programs sorted, it's time to begin your cardiovascular program. Below, you will find schedules for getting started in running, cycling, and swimming, but I devote the most time to getting started in running because it is the most likely to cause injury if performed incorrectly. However, with the right gradual progression you can still safely use running as your cardiovascular exercise and capitalize on running's greatest benefit: it burns the highest number of calories.

Starting From Zero Run Schedule

I know about starting from zero because this is the schedule I have used several times after taking a break from running while recovering from an injury. Before I started using periodization I would overtrain, get injured, stop running, get physical therapy, and then eventually start running again. It is a very slow progression. It is so intentionally, and I highly recommend following it if you are just beginning to run.

I know many people who have taken a break from running, or just decided one day to start running. Often, they run two miles; that feels great, so they go three miles the next run. They add another mile with each run, and they feel pretty good for the first two weeks, and then the injuries begin and they have to stop running, heal, and then start again.

It is best to use this schedule while running on a treadmill,

Starting Your Cardiovascular Program

because the platform has some flex, which absorbs shock. A treadmill also works well because it has the time display in big numbers right in front of you, allowing you to count your cadence and measure your times accurately. It is possible to do this progression outside on the sidewalk, but you will need a stopwatch, or some other way to time yourself.

This progression calls for three workouts a week, with a day off in between each workout. The run portions of the routine should be at an easy pace. This should be your beginning base pulse. This pace is one at which you can easily carry on a conversation. The five minutes of walking at the beginning and end of each session facilitate a proper warm-up and cool-down. Each workout should begin and end with proper stretching. Also, progress to the longer workouts each week only if everything feels good. That is to say, if you have tightness or soreness in a joint or muscle for two workouts in a row, treat it like an injury. See the chapters on deep tissue massage and icing. Once the issue is resolved, return to the progression, starting at the week prior to when the issue developed.

See the "Mechanics of Running" chapter for tips on proper form, or go to my website for more information on getting a Video Stride Analysis if you need more help.

When starting a new running program it is very important to get a new pair of shoes. Go to a running specialty store, like Future Track in Thousand Oaks, CA. Such stores are staffed by runners, who know how to help you select the right shoe. Many of these stores have treadmills that have video analysis, which can help determine if your foot strike has flaws that need to be corrected by shoes built to correct your specific issue.

New shoes are also important because they will absorb shock better than shoes that are worn out. The midsole of a running shoe is the layer between the insole and the outer sole. Our bodies are designed to run in bare feet on dirt and grass, which are very soft and they absorb a lot of shock. However, because most of us run mostly on much harder surfaces like asphalt and concrete, we need a soft and thick midsole in a shoe to mimic mother earth and absorb much of the shock. If you have mechanical issues in your stride, running in just any running shoe could cause issues. Many manufacturers design shoes to correct many common stride issues. The key is finding the right shoe, and the staff of a running specialty shop will be able to do that best.

"Natural Running Shoes," which have been the rage of late, can actually be very dangerous when running on hard surfaces. Again, going back to our original design, if you run mostly on dirt or grass, running shoes that have little or no padding or support may be okay. However, I caution against using these shoes on concrete and asphalt. Since they have no midsole to absorb shock, and concrete and asphalt will absorb only a small amount of shock, if any -- all of the shock generated when your feet touch the ground will be transmitted into you. This has been known to cause injury in even very experienced runners. So, wear a pair of real running shoes if you plan to run mostly on concrete and asphalt.

One good application I have seen for these minimalist shoes is during strength training. Because they don't have a midsole, they are actually more stable than most running shoes. In the gym, stability may be preferred over cushioning when strength training. However, I still just use an old pair of running shoes when I strength train.

With the right pair of new shoes, and being mindful of proper form, you are now ready to start running.

Starting Your Cardiovascular Program

The Schedule for the "Starting From Zero" Run Progression:

Run progression starting from "0" miles					
Week	Walk	Run	Walk	Run	Walk
1	5 mins	2 mins	2 mins	2 mins	5 mins
2	5 mins	3 mins	2 mins	3 mins	5 mins
3	5 mins	4 mins	2 mins	4 mins	5 mins
4	5 mins	2 mins	2 mins	2 mins	5 mins
5	5 mins	6 mins	2 mins	6 mins	5 mins
6	5 mins	7 mins	2 mins	7 mins	5 mins
7	5 mins	8 mins	2 mins	8 mins	5 mins
8	5 mins	5 mins	2 mins	5 mins	5 mins
9	5 mins	10 mins	2 mins	10 mins	5 mins
10	5 mins	12 mins	2 mins	12 mins	5 mins
11	5 mins	14 mins	2 mins	14 mins	5 mins
12	5 mins	10 mins	2 mins	10 mins	5 mins
13	5 mins	15 mins	2 mins	15 mins	5 mins
14	5 mins	30 mins			5 mins

After week 14, if all is well, you can start training for your first 5K using the schedule below. If you've come this far, I recommend finding a 5K race, which will coincide with the end of the peak phase. I think it is very important to have a race as a goal so you have something to work toward. I have often found during training that knowing I am on the hook for a race has served as motivation to complete a given workout with full energy. Also, keep in mind that the goal of running a race is not to win it, but simply to finish the race. By finishing the race you will have another marker by which to measure yourself when you finish the next periodization cycle. There is nothing more motivating than seeing the improvement resulting from your long-term commitment to yourself.

THE TRACK

To maximize your strength and speed, when using a running program which uses periodization, hills and track work will be incorporated in the peak phase. During track workouts is the only time I use a stopwatch. I use the stopwatch on the track because it allows me to precisely measure my pace. My pulse is still the biggest number on the display, and by keeping track of how fast I run each mile, I can see the improvement I make each week. I have found this to be highly motivating, as has everyone I have ever coached.

When I talk about running a mile on a track, I am actually referring to running 1600 meters, which is four laps, since most tracks today are 400 meters. This is actually a little longer than a mile, but because I am old school I still think of four laps as a mile.

Track workouts involve repeat miles. After stretching properly and running 1 mile at base pace as a warm-up, you will run 3 X 1-mile repeats. That is to say, you will run 1 mile at or near your AT, then walk 1 lap, then run another mile at or near AT, then walk 1 lap, then run 1 more mile at or near AT. To top-off your fuel supply, I recommend having one Accel Gel after running the first mile. After the last mile at pace, jog one more mile as a cool-down, and then stretch.

Each week you can expect to see times that are three to five seconds faster than the week before, while exerting the same effort. When you run on the track, the idea is to run at or near your AT. The improvement of three to five seconds a week documents your improved fitness. This improvement occurs because your legs have gotten stronger and your cardiovascular system has become more efficient. This means that if you run at the exact same tempo as the week before, you probably won't notice improvement. However, by using a HRM you may notice you will need to increase your tempo very slightly in order to get to your AT. Without the HRM, your improvements are imperceptible. Using a stopwatch with a HRM is the only way to map your improvement. The stopwatch provides the irrefutable evidence of your improved fitness and speed.

One more point about track work. Why do we run mile repeats and not 800s, or other distances? Many track coaches have long-distance runners run repeat half miles to improve "leg speed." For distance specialists, that is fine. However, what we are doing by running repeat miles is working on leg speed and also improving your cardiovascular system by improving your ability to run at or near your AT. To do this you must be at or near AT for more than a few seconds. It takes me about 800 meters to get my pulse to my AT. Accordingly, if I were to stop running at that point I would be training my muscles only to go faster. By running mile repeats, I am at or near my AT for another 800 meters, which means I am improving leg speed while also improving my body's ability to exert at that level. I am improving my body's ability to remove lactic acid and deliver oxygen and fuel better. This improved ability to deliver fuel and take away lactic acid is what leads to being able to run faster for longer.

HILLS

Hill runs are essential to build leg strength and improve mechanics. By running uphill, you are forced to lift your knees a little higher than during a stride on flat land. Anatomically, most of this is done by the iliopsoas, commonly known as the hip flexor. Once the foot is planted, the quadricep and gluteal muscle groups must work a little harder than when on flat terrain. Though most people hate running hills, you need to be committed to making them part of peak phase because they strengthen the most important muscles involved in running -- the big pushing muscles -- as well as your heart.

The key to running hills is similar to the key to track work: running at or near your AT for much of the run. Also, to the extent possible, hill running should be done on longer hills, which are medium grade. The hills I run near work are up to four miles long and medium grade, which allows me to settle into a pace near my AT and then hold that for the uphill portion of the run. Learning to run hills well will make you stronger, which will lead to faster times on the track and in races.

One of the best parts of running hills is that what goes up must come down. When done properly, running downhill can also improve your speed. Running downhill is best done with a shorter and controlled stride.

Since running hills is also about quality and not quantity, the higher the tempo you can maintain for the duration of the workout, the stronger and more fit you will become. That's why, when running hill workouts of more than five miles, I will take an Accel Gel between miles two and three.

5K RUNNING SCHEDULE

5K Running Periodization Schedule			
Base Phase - all runs are in base pulse range			
Week	Day 1	Day 2	Day 3
1	2 miles	2 miles	3 miles
2	3 miles	3 miles	4 miles
3	4 miles	4 miles	5 miles
4	2 miles	2 miles	3 miles
5	3 miles	3 miles	4 miles
6	4 miles	4 miles	5 miles
7	5 miles	5 miles	6 miles
8	3 miles	3 miles	4 miles
Building Phase - Day 1 and 2 runs are in building pulse range and Day 3 runs are in base pulse range			

STARTING YOUR CARDIOVASCULAR PROGRAM

Week	Day 1	Day 2	Day 3
9	2 miles	2 miles	4 miles
10	3 miles	3 miles	5 miles
11	4 miles	4 miles	6 miles
12	2 miles	2 miles	4 miles
13	3 miles	3 miles	5 miles
14	4 miles	4 miles	6 miles
15	5 miles	5 miles	7 miles
16	3 miles	3 miles	4 miles

Peak Phase - Day 1 and 2 runs are at or near AT, and Day 3 runs are in base pulse range. Day 1, mile repeats follow a proper stretch and a 1-mile base pace warm-up. After each mile run at or near AT, walk 1 lap. Day 2, hills are run at or near AT on the way up, and in your building pulse range on the way down.

Week	Day 1	Day 2	Day 3
17	2 X 1 mile repeats	2 miles hills	6 miles
18	3 X 1 mile repeats	3 miles hills	6 miles
19	3 X 1 mile repeats	4 miles hills	6 miles
20	2 X 1 mile repeats	2 miles hills	3 miles
21	3 X 1 mile repeats	3 miles hills	6 miles
22	3 X 1 mile repeats	4 miles hills	6 miles
23	3 X 1 mile repeats	5 miles hills	5 miles
24	1 X 1 mile repeats	2 miles hills	Race

After finishing the 24-week program, take a week off and then start base phase again. You may want to increase your mileage per workout a little and consider training for a 10K. Get a physical and compare the results to the numbers from your last physical. Think about getting a BLT or VO2 test to get your new pulse range numbers. You will likely find significant positive changes.

Running Race Pulse Protocol

Using a race pulse protocol is very helpful to bridle the "fresh" legs you will have from week 24, which will be a taper week. A "taper week" refers to the week preceding a race, during which you reduce, or taper, the amount of mileage you run. It is the same principle as a recovery week, which allows you to completely heal right before you race. With fresh legs and the normal amount of adrenaline you will have at the race start, you will tend to start the race too fast. Giving in to the adrenaline means you will go out way too fast, because you can, and then struggle for the rest of the race because you started the race way above your AT.

Before using a HRM, I always went out much too fast, and ran a really fast first mile, but then struggled for the rest of the race with mile splits that got slower. By going out too fast and just hanging on, I always had to endure a very high level of physical discomfort. By reaching or exceeding my AT way too early, my cardiovascular system was stuck. When I started using a HRM and this race pulse protocol, that all changed. Not only did I run faster races overall, even though my first mile was slower, I maintained a better overall pace and experienced a very manageable level of discomfort.

For anyone who wants to reach their genetic potential, some discomfort is involved, since exerting at that level during training is needed to cause adaptation, which will make you stronger. However, if reaching your genetic potential is less important than not experiencing a little discomfort, then you probably don't need to use this protocol, but I would recommend you continue to use this overall program.

So, for those who want to find their genetic potential, the first component of developing a race pulse protocol is knowing your AT. From this number, we will work backward to the start of the race. Although the run training program calls for you to train during the peak phase at or near your AT, the only time you want to be at your AT when you race is during the last mile or two. This is because, since you will be at your AT by definition, it is not a sustainable pace for more than a mile or two.

Accordingly, and using my AT of 175 as an example, I run the first mile of a 5K at about 170 beats per minute (BPM). Often, because I respond well to taper weeks and my legs heal and feel fresh, I usually feel like I am jogging. The truth is, I am usually running times in the first mile of a race that are very close to the times I run on the track in training. It just feels slow, because my legs are fresh.

During the second mile, I let the pulse creep up to 172 to 173 and settle into a good rhythm. Then, during the last mile, I go to 175. With half a mile to go, if I feel good I will begin to press and let my pulse creep up to 178 or so, and if there is someone I want to chase down I will kick it into my top gear, especially when I can see the finish line. When doing this, I have seen my pulse climb as high as 200. The pulse I will run during the last mile is not sustainable, but because I will run at that level at the end of the race, it is not an issue. By following a smart race pulse protocol, I not only reduce the amount of stress I feel created by a fear of bonking, I have continued to get a little faster each time I race.

19. Getting Started on the Bike

ONE OF THE MOST IMPORTANT PARTS OF GETTING STARTED ON THE bike is to realize that your "sit bones" (ischial tuberosity) located at the bottom of your pelvis, will likely be more sore than your leg muscles. Your "sit bones" will need to adapt before you will be able to ride longer distances in comfort. Having the right seat is the best way to reduce any discomfort. Also, more padding is not necessarily better. More padding can fill in and around the sit bones and possibly press on nerves in the region, which will only make you more uncomfortable. For many, the best solution will be to get the right seat, and follow the schedule below. To determine the right seat, see your local bike dealer.

Also, depending on weather and what time of day you will be riding, a good spin class can be a great substitute for riding on the road. During my first winter of riding I found myself in a great spin class in Washington DC, taught by a semi-pro female cyclist. She taught me I could climb well beyond what I thought I could. Additionally, while a spin class can be great because you are with other people, most spin classes work you at very high loads and tempos, which means they may be best placed in building and peak phases.

However, when getting started, you should be riding at a tempo which allows you to easily carry on a conversation, so a better option may be to spend some time on a stationary bike that is not in a spin class. Also, as discussed earlier, you want a cadence which is right around 90 for maximum efficiency. So, if your bike does not have a cadence monitor, you can buy a small computer for your bike. The simplest cost less than $100 and will measure speed, cadence, and time, which are all the data sets you really need.

GETTING STARTED ON THE BIKE SCHEDULE

Getting Started Bike Schedule			
Week	Day 1	Day 2	Day 3
1	20 mins	20 mins	30 mins
2	25 mins	25 mins	40 mins
3	30 mins	30 mins	50 mins
4	20 mins	20 mins	30 mins
5	35 mins	35 mins	60 mins
6	40 mins	40 mins	70 mins
7	45 mins	45 mins	80 mins
8	30 mins	30 mins	50 mins
9	50 mins	50 mins	90 mins
10	55 mins	55 mins	100 mins
11	60 mins	60 mins	110 mins
12	40 mins	40 mins	65 mins

Now you are ready to start some group rides. Most bike shops have a variety of group rides. You can also join a cycling club for group rides. Group rides are a great way to get a good workout in, and make new friends who are also fitness-minded. Most cycling clubs also have partnerships with local bike shops and they provide discounts to club members. Given the addictive nature of this sport, coupled with all the cool clothing and other gear you will want, getting 10% off will add up.

If you want to maximize your speed, like running, you will need to do interval and hill work. If you followed the above Getting Started Bike Schedule your base conditioning should be set and you can go right to the Building Phase of the schedule below. If you are already a veteran cyclist, but you have never used periodization, start with the Base Phase below.

Similar to the 5K Running Schedule above, the program below is designed to increase muscle strength and speed while also enhancing your cardiovascular development through interval and hill workouts in the building and peak phases. I recommend getting a VO2 or BLT test done at the end of week 12 to identify your new building and peak phase pulse ranges. Not only should you expect to see pulse improvements over time; you should also expect to see your power output increase in those ranges. Since you will be doing the tests on a bike, the watts metric can be measured. These new tests should provide numbers, which will record your improvements, guide your next phases of training, and also serve as great motivation to "stay on the program."

FULL PERIODIZATION 24-WEEK CYCLING PROGRAM

Full Cycling Periodization Program			
Base Phase - all rides are in base pulse range.			
Week	Day 1	Day 2	Day 3
1	10 miles	10 miles	20 miles
2	15 miles	15 miles	25 miles
3	20 miles	20 miles	30 miles
4	10 miles	10 miles	20 miles
5	15 miles	15 miles	25 miles
6	20 miles	20 miles	30 miles
7	20 miles	20 miles	35 miles
8	10 miles	10 miles	25 miles

Building Phase - Day 1 and 2 rides: the first number is the number of miles in building pulse (BP) followed by the number of miles of recovery (R) between each interval, which is easy pedaling. These rides should include a 5-to-10-minute warm-up and cool-down in base pulse range. (T) indicates the total number of miles for that workout. Day 3 rides are in base pulse range. So, for example, using week 9, Day 1, following stretching and warm-up, ride 1 mile in Building Pulse, recover for 1 mile with easy pedaling, and repeat until you have ridden 10 miles. Day 2 is the same, and Day 3 is 25 miles at Base Pulse.

Week	Day 1	Day 2	Day 3
9	1 BP/1 R/T 10	1 BP/1 R/T 10	25 miles
10	2 BP/2 R/T 15	2 BP/2 R/T 15	30 miles
11	2 BP/1 R/T 15	2 BP/1 R/T 15	35 miles
12	1 BP/1 R/T 10	1 BP/1 R/T 10	25 miles
13	2 BP/2 R/T 15	2 BP/2 R/T 15	30 miles
14	2 BP/1 R/T 15	2 BP/1 R/T 15	35 miles
15	3 BP/1 R/T 20	3 BP/1 R/T 20	40 miles
16	1 BP/1 R/T 10	1 BP/1 R/T 10	25 miles

Peak Phase - Day 1 rides should be in hills at or near your AT when climbing. Group rides make a great environment to work hard when climbing. Day 2 rides are intervals and the first number is the number of miles at or near AT, followed by the number of recovery (R) miles or easy pedaling, followed by (T) which indicates the total miles for the ride. All rides should include a 5-to-10-minute warm-up and cool-down in base pulse range. Day 3 rides are in base pulse range.

Week	Day 1	Day 2	Day 3
17	20-30 miles	1 AT/1 R/T 10	25 miles
18	20-30 miles	2 AT/2 R/T 15	30 miles
19	20-30 miles	2 AT/1 R/T 15	35 miles
20	10-20 miles	1 AT/1 R/T 10	25 miles
21	20-30 miles	2 AT/2 R/T 15	40 miles
22	20-30 miles	2 AT/1 R/T 15	45 miles
23	20-30 miles	3 AT/1 R/T 20	50 miles
24	10-20 miles	1 AT/1 R/T 10	Race

After finishing the 24-week program, take a week off and then start base phase again. You may want to increase your mileage per workout a little. Get a physical and compare it to the numbers from your last physical. Think about getting a BLT or VO2 test. You will likely find significant positive changes.

20. Getting Started Swimming

BECAUSE SWIMMING IS SO FORM-DEPENDENT, AND BECAUSE there is so much to be gained with proper form, you may want to join a master's swim team or club. If you go this route, you won't need the table below, as the team or club coach will provide you with workouts. Just make sure the coach knows you are new to swimming and should keep an eye on you so he or she can give you some tips on how to improve your stroke. Master's swim team regulars usually don't get much form coaching, since most of them have swim backgrounds, or have been swimming for a long time, so the coach's job is to give them a workout and let them swim.

As a new swimmer, you will likely need a substantial amount of help. The amount of help you need may exceed the coach's ability during group swims, since he or she will have multiple lanes of swimmers to manage. Most coaches will allow you to pay them a small fee for one-on-one coaching sessions, outside of the regular swim team workouts. This will likely be money well-spent.

Also, if you are a new swimmer, there is some pool protocol you will need to be mindful of. These protocols serve both safety and courtesy, helping to maintain peace in the pool.

If there are already swimmers in all the lanes, find a lane that has swimmers of similar ability to yours. It's not courteous or safe to just jump in and start swimming. Once you have identified the right lane, walk to the edge of the pool and stand in front of the lane. When the other swimmers reach the end and are right in front of you, they should acknowledge you. Ask if you can join them. If you will be the second person to swim in the lane, it is traditional to "split" the lane. This means you will swim back and forth on one side of the lane and the other person will stay on the other side of the lane. However, if your addition to the lane means more than two people will be in the lane, you will need to agree to swim in a "circle." Usually, swimming in a circle means swimming in a counter-clockwise pattern. This allows more than two swimmers to use the lane without running into each other.

If you join other swimmers in a lane, you should wait about five seconds to follow the swimmer in front of you. If you catch the swimmer in front of you before reaching the end of the pool, you can either pass them, if the lane is wide enough, or at the turn you can ask if it is okay if you go in front of them. The same is true in reverse. If the swimmer who is following you turns out to be faster than you, they will normally touch your toes to let you know they are there. If this happens, don't be concerned; just offer to let them go in front of you at the turn. After a few laps, if you find yourself in a lane with swimmers who are much faster than you and you are constantly getting in someone's way, move to a slower lane.

For swimming gear, you may want to buy a set of fins, a pull buoy, a kick board, and a snorkel. I like to warm up and cool down by swimming freestyle easy for a few hundred yards. Easy freestyle for most beginners means you will be going pretty slowly and your legs will likely sink, even though you are kicking. Sinking legs is not just about swimming slowly; it is also usually the result of weak core muscles.

To help strengthen the specific core muscles, which will help promote better body position, I use a snorkel, fins, and a kick board after warming up. With the kick board fully extended, I breathe through the snorkel while looking at the bottom of the pool. I keep the board still and rotate slightly at the waist and my heels come just above the surface of the water. If your feet come out of the water and make a big splash, you need to adjust your kick so the top of your heel is the only part of your foot that breaks the surface of the water. I do this kicking technique as part of my warm-up for 200 meters.

As covered earlier, if you are just starting to swim, don't expect to be able to swim for very long during the first few months. When I started, I could swim only 25 meters and then I had to stop for at least 30 seconds to catch my breath. The first day I swam a total of 100 meters (m). It took me three months before I could swim 200 meters without stopping. Swimming will require the most patience, because improvement will be the most gradual.

After you have been swimming for a few months, test yourself. The test consists of swimming 100m three times, with 20 seconds of rest. If you are still out of breath with 20 seconds of rest, take 30. The idea is to swim as fast as you can and have no more variance than five seconds between each 100m. So, if you swam the first 100m in 1:45, the second in 1:55, and the last one in 2:00, the variance would be 15 seconds, which is too much. To correct this, next time swim the first 100m a little slower and see if you can swim all three between 1:50 and 1:55, a five-second variance. Do this test once a month and note your times in your journal. Over time you should notice not only that your swim times get faster; you will also be able to cut the rest intervals (RI). Also, if during the first weeks the RIs are too short, make them as long as they need to be so you can get through the workout. As you get stronger, you will be able to shorten them.

Getting Started Swim Schedule

Getting Started Swim Schedule			
Week	Day 1	Day 2	Day 3
1	10 X 25m, 20 RI	10 X 25m, 20 RI	10 X 25m, 20 RI
2	12 X 25m, 20 RI	12 X 25m, 20 RI	12 X 25m, 20 RI
3	14 X 25m, 20 RI	14 X 25m, 20 RI	14 X 25m, 20 RI
4	10 X 25m, 20 RI	10 X 25m, 20 RI	10 X 25m, 20 RI
5	5 X 50m, 25 RI	5 X 50m, 25 RI	5 X 25m, 25 RI
6	6 X 50m, 25 RI	6 X 50m, 25 RI	6 X 50m, 25 RI
7	7 X 50m, 25 RI	7 X 50m, 25 RI	7 X 50m, 25 RI
8	5 X 50m, 25 RI	5 X 50m, 25 RI	5 X 50m, 25 RI
9	4 X 100m, 30 RI	4 X 100m, 30 RI	4 X 100m, 30 RI
10	5 X 100m, 30 RI	5 X 100m, 30 RI	3 X 200m, 45 RI
11	6 X 100m, 30 RI	6 X 100m, 30 RI	4 X 200m, 45 RI
12	4 X 100m, 30 RI	4 X 100m, 30 RI	3 X 200m, 45 RI

21. Logging

I THINK IT IS A GREAT IDEA TO KEEP A LOG OR DIARY OF YOUR training, especially if you are just starting a program. Logs serve as great reminders of what you did when, and they map your progress. Again, the best motivation is knowing that you are improving.

Also, if you have trouble remembering each weight you use for the many strength-training exercises, use a daily exercise log. Go to my website for more information on a daily log you can use. To be clear, a daily log is different from your long-term diary. The daily log is to remind you of the amount of weight and number of repetitions you used last time, while a diary is meant to record the general nature of your workouts.

A long-term diary will serve as a history of what you have done over a period of time and help identify positive or negative trends in your fitness program. If you have a particularly good or bad workout or race, you can look at the conditions preceding the workout or race and likely identify the cause. I still use a diary in this way regarding cycling and swimming, since I am new to these sports. I have been trying different workout sequences the week before I race and then look at my race results. Over the last couple of years, I have been able to get a feel for the exact taper that works best for me.

The key to keeping a long-term diary is the same as the key to the rest of this program: keep it simple. I would suggest that you record your weight, the amount of sleep you get each night, and the type of training you do each day. You might want to record your swim "test" times, repeat mile times on the track, and your times for certain high-exertion bike rides, so you can see your progress over time.

Stay away from trying to capture each parameter of each workout, since that is too much data and it won't really tell you much from day to day.

Record the important numbers in your peak phase, keep an eye on the scale, get a VO2 test or BLT periodically, and a physical annually to map your progress.

22. Final Word

THE DIFFERENT PROGRAMS IN THIS BOOK MAY BE A LITTLE OVERwhelming to understand and use all at one time. However, I have simplified each area as much as possible by stripping away much of the extraneous information, leaving only the information you need to make adjustments, and understand why.

So, if you can only initiate the eating program, because you have not found the time to start working out yet, then do just that. When you have lost some weight and want to start sculpting your body, start with finding 1 hour a day, during 4 days in a week. Start by doing strength training for 30 minutes followed by 30 minutes of cardiovascular exercise during those 4 days. When you have worked this into your life and you like the results you are seeing, look for additional time and consider lengthening the cardiovascular part of your program.

The idea is to understand your body and what you are doing to it. Hopefully, by reading this book you will have a better understanding. The challenge is to make a decision to bring smart change to improve your fitness and health, which will in turn improve your quality of life. By phasing these changes into your life gradually, you will find that your quality and balance of life improve.

The goal in writing this book was to help impart what I have learned about health and fitness, so you might also benefit from those lessons.

I am blessed and lead a very happy and full life. I am in balance because I have a wonderful family that comes first, then work, and then play. I am also smart about all of it and how I prioritize my time. I will admit that I have a lot of full days, but as animals we are born to be active, and I have a lot of fun with my family, at work and at play.

If you also consider that most of the worst diseases in the world can be prevented simply through improved fitness and health, we should all be making time to be fit and healthy. My wish is that you will use the knowledge in this book to improve your health and fitness and lead a longer, happier life. So, train smart and have fun.

Appendix A

Lab and EKG results from my 2012 physical examination:

TESTS	RESULT	FLAG	UNITS	REFERENCE INTERVAL	LAB
CMP14+LP+3AC+CBC/D/Plt+TSH					
Chemistries					
Glucose, Serum	90		mg/dL	65-99	01
Uric Acid, Serum	4.6		mg/dL	3.7-8.6	01
Therapeutic target for gout patients: <6.0					
BUN	19		mg/dL	6-24	01
Creatinine, Serum	0.86		mg/dL	0.76-1.27	01
eGFR If NonAfricn Am	100		mL/min/1.73	>59	01
eGFR If Africn Am	116		mL/min/1.73	>59	01
Note: A persistent eGFR <60 mL/min/1.73 m2 (3 months or more) may indicate chronic kidney disease. An eGFR >59 mL/min/1.73 m2 with an elevated urine protein also may indicate chronic kidney disease. Calculated using CKD-EPI formula.					
BUN/Creatinine Ratio	22	High		9-20	01
Sodium, Serum	141		mmol/L	134-144	01
Potassium, Serum	4.0		mmol/L	3.5-5.2	01
Chloride, Serum	102		mmol/L	97-108	01
Carbon Dioxide, Total	26		mmol/L	20-32	01
Calcium, Serum	8.9		mg/dL	8.7-10.2	01
Phosphorus, Serum	3.8		mg/dL	2.5-4.5	01
Protein, Total, Serum	6.1		g/dL	6.0-8.5	01
Albumin, Serum	4.4		g/dL	3.5-5.5	01
Globulin, Total	1.7		g/dL	1.5-4.5	01
A/G Ratio	2.6	High		1.1-2.5	01
Bilirubin, Total	0.3		mg/dL	0.0-1.2	01
Alkaline Phosphatase, S	70		IU/L	25-150	01
LDH	252	High	IU/L	0-225	01
AST (SGOT)	33		IU/L	0-40	01
ALT (SGPT)	27		IU/L	0-55	01
Lipids					01

FINAL REPORT

Fit at 50: Back From the Brink, Naturally

TESTS	RESULT	FLAG	UNITS	REFERENCE INTERVAL	LAB
Cholesterol, Total	191		mg/dL	100-199	01
Triglycerides	73		mg/dL	0-149	01
HDL Cholesterol	81		mg/dL	>39	01
According to ATP-III Guidelines, HDL-C >59 mg/dL is considered a negative risk factor for CHD.					
LDL Cholesterol Calc	95		mg/dL	0-99	01
T. Chol/HDL Ratio	2.4		ratio units	0.0-5.0	01
Thyroid					01
TSH	1.520		uIU/mL	0.450-4.500	01
CBC, Platelet Ct, and Diff					01
WBC	7.4		x10E3/uL	4.0-10.5	01
RBC	4.60		x10E6/uL	4.10-5.60	01
Hemoglobin	14.2		g/dL	12.5-17.0	01
Hematocrit	42.5		%	36.0-50.0	01
MCV	92		fL	80-98	01
MCH	30.9		pg	27.0-34.0	01
MCHC	33.4		g/dL	32.0-36.0	01
RDW	13.0		%	11.7-15.0	01
Platelets	222		x10E3/uL	140-415	01
Neutrophils	70		%	40-74	01
Lymphs	20		%	14-46	01
Monocytes	8		%	4-13	01
Eos	2		%	0-7	01
Basos	0		%	0-3	01
Neutrophils (Absolute)	5.2		x10E3/uL	1.8-7.8	01
Lymphs (Absolute)	1.5		x10E3/uL	0.7-4.5	01
Monocytes (Absolute)	0.6		x10E3/uL	0.1-1.0	01
Eos (Absolute)	0.1		x10E3/uL	0.0-0.4	01
Baso (Absolute)	0.0		x10E3/uL	0.0-0.2	01
Immature Granulocytes	0		%	0-2	01
Immature Grans (Abs)	0.0		x10E3/uL	0.0-0.1	01
Prostate-Specific Ag, Serum					

APPENDIX A

	Patient ID	Control Number	Account Number	Account Phone Number	Biz	
MCLAUGHLIN			Account Address			
MATTHEW						
Patient Sex	Patient Phone	Total Volume				
Age (Y/M/D)	Date of Birth	Sex				
	Patient Address		Add'l Local Information			
				UPIN:		
Date and Time Collected 04/17/12 16:39	Date Entered 04/18/12	Date and Time Reported 04/18/12 14:13ET	Physicians Name	NPI	Physician ID	

TESTS	RESULT	FLAG	UNITS	REFERENCE INTERVAL	LAB
Prostate Specific Ag, Serum	0.7		ng/mL	0.0-4.0	01

Roche ECLIA methodology.

According to the American Urological Association, Serum PSA should decrease and remain at undetectable levels after radical prostatectomy. The AUA defines biochemical recurrence as an initial PSA value 0.2 ng/mL or greater followed by a subsequent confirmatory PSA value 0.2 ng/mL or greater.
Values obtained with different assay methods or kits cannot be used interchangeably. Results cannot be interpreted as absolute evidence of the presence or absence of malignant disease.

MCLAUGHLIN, MATTHEW
04/18/12 02:16   FINAL REPORT

Fit at 50: Back From the Brink, Naturally

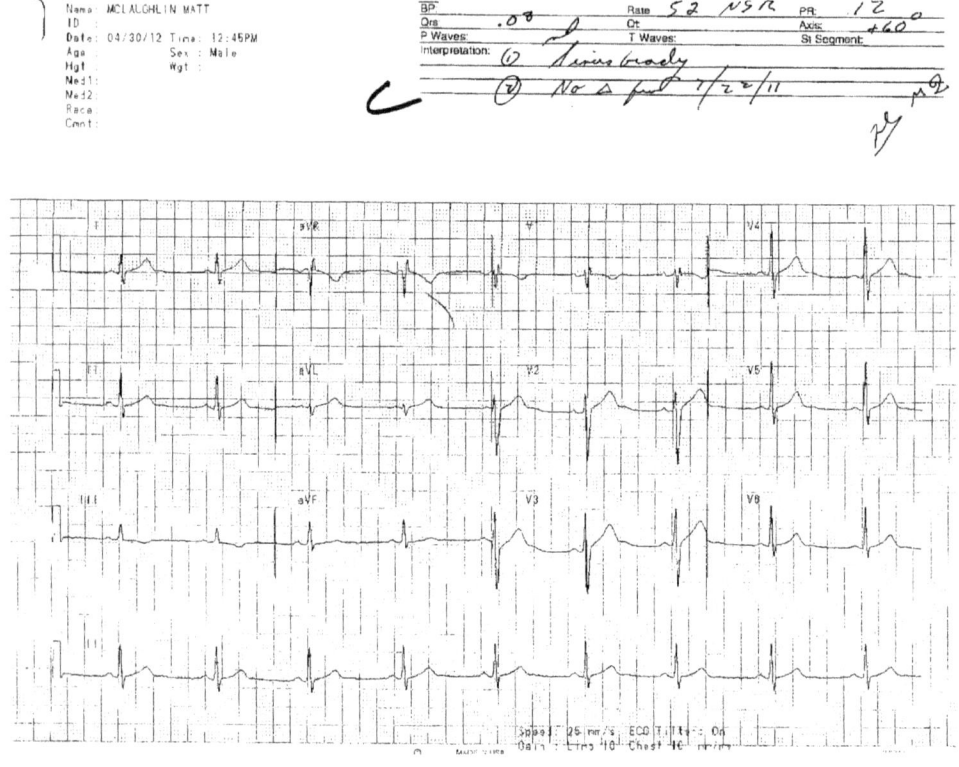

References

Bompa, Tudor O. PhD, *Periodization Training for Sports,* Champaign, IL, Human Kinetics, 1999

Burke, Edmond R. PhD, *Optimal Muscle Recovery: Your Guide to Achieving Peak Physical Performance,* Garden City Park, NY, Avery Publishing Group, 1999

Ivy, John, PhD and Portman, Robert, PhD, *The Performance Zone,* North Bergen, NJ, Basic Health Publications, Inc, 2004

Janssen, Peter, MD, *Lactate Threshold Training,* Champaign, IL, Human Kinetics, 2001

Kreider, Richard B., Fry, Andrew C. and O'Toole, Mary L., *Overtraining in Sports,* Champaign, IL, Human Kinetics, 1998

Powers, Scott K. and Howley, Edward T., *Exercise Physiology, Theory and Application to Fitness and Performance. Fifth Edition*, New York, NY, McGraw-Hill, 2004.

CPSIA information can be obtained
at www.ICGtesting.com
Printed in the USA
JSHW011237090423
40097JS00003B/10